THE
NORDIC GUIDE
TO LIVING
10 YEARS LONGER

• •

10 EASY TIPS TO LIVE
A HEALTHIER, HAPPIER LIFE

DR BERTIL MARKLUND

Translation by Stuart Tudball

piatkus

PIATKUS

First published in Great Britain in 2017 by Piatkus
Originally published in Swedish under the title *10 Tips* by Volante AB, Sweden

Copyright © Bertil Marklund 2017

English translation © Stuart Tudball 2017
Published in agreement with Ahlander Agency

1 3 5 7 9 10 8 6 4 2

A CIP catalogue record for this book
is available from the British Library.

ISBN 978-0-349-41540-6

Typeset in Sabon by M Rules
Printed and bound in Great Britain by
Clays Ltd, St Ives plc

Papers used by Piatkus are from well-managed forests
and other responsible sources.

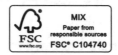

Piatkus
An imprint of
Little, Brown Book Group
Carmelite House
50 Victoria Embankment
London EC4Y 0DZ

An Hachette UK Company
www.hachette.co.uk

www.improvementzone.co.uk

Disclaimer
The information in this book will be relevant to the majority of people but may not
be applicable in each individual case so it is advised that professional medical advice
is obtained for specific health matters. The author and publisher disclaim any liability
directly or indirectly from the use of material in this book by any person.

Contents

Introduction

● ● ● ● ● ● ● ● ● ● ● ● ● ● ● ● ● ● ● ●

I've spent a lot of time over the years thinking about how one should live one's life in order to have as much time on this earth as possible. Both of my parents had multiple risk factors and unfortunately I lost them far too early. That shook me up. Would their genes also have a negative impact on my health and longevity? So I decided to get to the bottom of what I needed to do to enjoy as long and healthy a life as possible.

I am a physician with over twenty years' experience in clinical patient care and I have treated countless patients throughout the years. I have also done extensive research in areas such as family medicine and public health for more than twenty years. As a doctor and researcher, I had access to all the research I needed and, of course, I was already quite well informed about the issues. In the medical world we talk a lot about risk factors that lead to disease and premature death. However, I began to think along new lines and became increasingly interested in the health promotion perspective – how to boost health rather than focusing on disease and death. I decided to study health factors instead of risk factors, to shift from the negative to the positive, with a focus on new knowledge about why some people are so healthy and live so long.

The research showed me what I wanted to know – how to stay healthy and live longer. Studies showed that the genetic component only accounts for around 25 per cent of longevity, with lifestyle coming in at 75 per cent. The figures may vary somewhat between studies, but they all indicate that lifestyle is the critical factor. This was a relatively new finding, and I was pleased to learn that I was the one in control of my longevity, not my genes. I can affect my health by shaping my own lifestyle and the benefits are fantastic – potentially adding as many as ten healthy years, maybe more, to my life. It is up to me to decide how I want to age – and don't want to age.

Sweden is one of the healthiest countries in the world and in all of the Nordic countries there is increasing awareness of the importance of living a healthy lifestyle. However, the themes in this book are wholly universal and can be applied to anyone seeking to make a change in their life. I want to pass on what I've learned about lifestyle changes for a healthy and long life to everyone interested in improving and boosting their health and putting the brake on disease and ageing. Hopefully this little book will help you. It can be summed up as a short guide to a long life.

WHY YET ANOTHER SELF-HELP BOOK?

There is already a plethora of self-help books on all sorts of health conditions and lifestyle choices, how to make yourself feel better. People tend to buy books about something in their lives that they want to change and that book is often 300–400 pages long, sometimes even more. If you're really ambitious you might read the whole book in less than a week or so. The content is good, the advice plentiful, but the problem is that as you reach the end of the book there is a considerable risk that you'll feel completely overwhelmed. There is so much to absorb that you have to take deep breaths before you begin putting the new advice into practice.

There is a big gap between words and action – and that is a problem.

The changes you are willing to make straight away, preferably the same day or the day after, have a great chance of success. If you start thinking that you have to work yourself up to it and then begin early next week or maybe next month, then there is a major chance that there will be no change. Instead, after a while you might find yourself buying a new self-help book in the hope that it will offer some easier options.

But this book is different and I'll tell you why.

Nordic focus

The Nordic countries are known for their pared-down simplicity, and in Sweden, we refer to this as *lagom*. There is no English equivalent to this inherently Swedish word, but it is best translated as 'just the right amount,' and in Sweden we often say, 'just the right amount is best'. *Lagom* can be applied to almost any situation – from the amount of coffee you'd like to how much exercise you should do – but more than that, it indicates balance and a Swedish idea of moderation. *The Nordic Guide to Living 10 Years Longer* applies this ethos to health – and it is important for me to express that to live a healthy life, you do not have to go to extremes. It's the small and simple changes that amount to a happier, healthier life.

Creates motivation

It is important to have an answer to the question of *why* you should change your lifestyle. The answer is that it gives you a chance to live ten years longer, and be healthier with it, and this is hopefully a strong motivator to make a lifestyle change. Most people would want a longer and healthier life and the basis of this book is to explain how you can achieve that.

Rooted in expert knowledge

All the facts and tips in this book are based on the experience and knowledge I've gained over the years, as a doctor in primary care and as a researcher in general medicine and public health. The book's facts are also founded on extensive studies of scientific literature, health research and statements by health experts.

New knowledge about inflammation

This guide is based on exciting research showing that the big threat to our health is the occurrence of inflammation in the body. The common thread running through the book is how this happens, the consequences it has and how we can protect ourselves against it.

Promotion and prevention

This book is built around two different perspectives. It provides suggestions on health promotion activities that you can do to feel good and stay feeling good – measures that lead to a healthy life. At the same time, it also explains how these measures will help you to stave off ill health.

Health is not a static state. We all shuttle between good health and ill health throughout our life.

But health, like life, is complex. You can feel good despite having a disease while a physically fit person can experience ill health and feel bad. We are all born different, but everyone can still do something for their health.

A health promotion perspective starts by looking at what creates and contributes to good health. This approach also involves accepting that there is no single factor that leads to health – there are numerous contributory factors and they are all interdependent, hence the ten chapters in this book. The key is to activate the inherent powers that we all have in order to achieve meaningful, longer and healthier lives – and not just to achieve good health in itself, but because good health is a resource that will help you achieve other goals in life such as travelling or spending time with family and friends.

This book gives advice on making the body and soul feel good. And this advice is for everyone. If you already feel good, you can reinforce and retain that feeling. And if you're already suffering ill health or disease, there is advice that can boost aspects of your lifestyle and help you move from ill health to health, or keep your health from deteriorating further.

PLENTY OF SIMPLE ADVICE – TAKE THAT FIRST STEP

The most important, but perhaps also most difficult, thing is to take the first step towards changing your lifestyle. So choose something that is relatively easy to change and get started now. Then use this book for support and as a reference to help you add more new habits to your life one step at a time. The transition to a healthy lifestyle shouldn't be a chore – it should feel positive and meaningful. That way you will stick to these new habits for the future. See yourself eating well, see yourself cycling up that long hill. It is important to create positive images of what is going to happen – this increases the chance of it becoming a reality.

Keep returning to the book, discuss it with your friends, share your top tips. This keeps the idea of health positivity alive.

What determines the length of your life?

• • • • • • • • • • • • • • • • • • •

As I mentioned in the introduction, we now know that your lifestyle is the most significant factor for a long and healthy life. You are very much able to influence your longevity and your health through active choices.

HOW MANY YEARS CAN LIFE ACTUALLY BE EXTENDED BY?

Different healthy lifestyle changes can give different outcomes. The figures mentioned in the book are averages for everyone involved in a particular study. This means that if a change in lifestyle has given an average of seven more years of life for all those in the study, the number of years for the individuals in the group may vary from three to eleven, for example. There is no real way of knowing exactly what the outcome will be in each individual case due to the fact that each person has their own state of health, but the message is still clear: making this lifestyle change increases the chance of improving health and extending life by a number of years.

One thing to note, however, is that if you make several lifestyle changes, you can't simply add up all the years of extended life for each particular change. Instead, the effects merge into each other, further increasing the likelihood of delaying diseases, feeling healthy and extending your life.

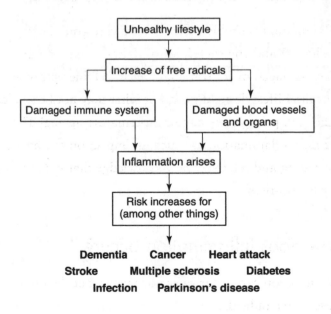

Figure 1. An unhealthy lifestyle leads to increased risk of disease

Before we begin with advice for good health, we first need to understand how things fit together. How can we build up and strengthen our body and mental health so that we can feel good and protect ourselves against inflammation?

INFLAMMATION – THE BIG THREAT

The big threat to our health is the occurrence of inflammation in the body, largely due to an unhealthy lifestyle. I'll be showing how lifestyle and inflammation are connected, how they affect our health and how we can avoid it.

Inflammation is problematic because you won't know you have it and you therefore won't know that you are being damaged by it. You might even feel fine with your unhealthy lifestyle right now, but what may not be so clear is the high price you're paying – premature ageing! The fact that inflammation has such an impact on our health is fascinating and relatively new knowledge that not everyone may be aware of.

How does inflammation occur?

Inflammation can occur in various ways, but the main cause is free radicals.

When we breathe in, oxygen enters our lungs, transfers to the blood system and is carried off to all the cells in the body. The cells then use the oxygen to produce energy for their critical functions. This process forms a by-product, called free radicals. The body is able to use small amounts of free radicals, but an unhealthy lifestyle creates too many. These electrically charged substances then go on the rampage, damaging cells in the body and causing inflammation. All cells are vulnerable to damage, in tissues, blood vessels and various organs. Our immune system also suffers (see figure 1).

What does long-term inflammation cause?

As we age, the damage and inflammation caused by free radicals becomes clearer. The immune system fails and bacteria, viruses and cancer cells are able to multiply and spread. But damage to the immune system can also make it over-ambitious so that it starts attacking the body's own normal cells. This gives rise to what are known as autoimmune diseases such as rheumatic pain, psoriasis and inflammatory bowel disease.

Long-term inflammation also means that the body's tissues, blood vessels and organs have sustained damage and their function will gradually deteriorate. Overall, inflammation can lead to a number of different diseases, including those named in figure 1.

Many of our most common diseases have the same root cause: inflammation.

HOW TO BOOST YOUR HEALTH AND COMBAT INFLAMMATION

Choosing a healthy lifestyle boosts your health while also stimulating the self-healing processes which, in various ways, combat the occurrence and harmful effects of inflammation. You decide, through your lifestyle, which path you want to take towards better health.

1. Build up a powerful immune system through a health-promoting and invigorating lifestyle

2. Reduce the production of free radicals through a preventive lifestyle

3. Render the free radicals harmless through a protective lifestyle

13

Build up a powerful immune system

Your immune system comprises your lymph glands, spleen and bone marrow, plus a large number of white blood cells of various kinds that patrol the body on the hunt for intruders. They defend the body against external invasion by finding and destroying harmful bacteria and viruses. They also deal with and kill off the body's cells that have been damaged by free radicals and that risk transforming into cancer cells.

A particular type of white blood cell known as 'natural killers' or 'NK cells' are the immune system's special forces. As soon as they discover an intruder, they try to make cell-to-cell contact and release a toxin that forces its way into the alien cell and destroys it. That's how fantastic our body is.

We also have a large and developed immune system in the mucous membranes of the intestines, which works in partnership with the bacteria there. Foreign objects enter our body all the time as we eat and drink, and the gut's immune system can distinguish between what is harmful and what is beneficial for our health. Good food and low levels of stress are two ways to create a strong immune system in the gut.

Choosing a healthy lifestyle enables us to build up strong immune defences. The number of immune cells can be increased, along with their activity levels. This ensures that we are well equipped to resist infections and the development of cancer.

Reduce the production of free radicals

A healthy lifestyle means living in a way that significantly reduces the production of free radicals and thus also reduces the damage to our immune system, blood vessels and organs. This in turn reduces inflammation and consequently also the risk of contracting a range of different diseases (see figure 2 below). This book describes how a healthy lifestyle can seriously reduce the number of free radicals.

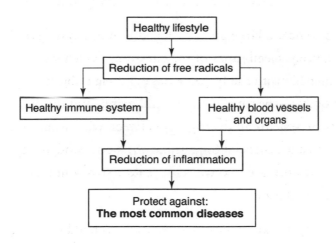

Figure 2. A healthy lifestyle protects against the most common diseases

Smoking – by far the most significant cause of free radicals and inflammation

Smoking is one of the worst choices you can make if you want to enjoy a long and healthy life. Smoking significantly increases the occurrence of free radicals, which directly damage our blood vessels, immune system and organs. In short, smoking leads to increased inflammation in the body.

The smoke also contains carcinogenic substances, which result in a greater incidence of lung disease, cardiovascular disease, cancer and a whole host of other diseases. Smoking thus speeds up our ageing, with research showing that smokers lose eight to twelve years of their life on average.

Imagine being a smoker who stops smoking and instead starts living a healthier life. Since the body is able to gradually recover, you could find yourself going from minus eight years of life expectancy to maybe eight plus years, potentially giving you an increased lifespan of sixteen years and a healthier life at that! Perhaps knowing this can provide the motivation to take that positive leap to stop smoking.

Render the free radicals harmless

The body has developed protection against attack from free radicals, in the form of antioxidants. Since the production of antioxidants in our body begins to tail off around the age of twenty-five, these need to be added via our food. More about that on page 62.

IMPROVE YOUR HEALTH – START TODAY!

If you have or have had an unhealthy lifestyle, forget what you did before. The important thing is what you do now, tomorrow and for the rest of your life. The rejuvenating and healing process kicks in as soon as your lifestyle changes for the better and the effects are quick to take hold. This is true whenever you choose to start something new – in other words, it's never too late. It doesn't matter what you begin with, the important thing is that you do something that has a positive impact on your health.

The result will be a healthier and longer life.

Research shows

A major study conducted in eleven European countries over the course of twelve years reported dramatic results: a reduction in cancer mortality of 60 per cent over the period of the study among people who switched to a healthier lifestyle.

The researchers also drew the conclusion that those who lived a healthier life worked out to be fourteen years younger in biological terms over the whole length of the study.

THE GOAL OF THIS BOOK

In this book, I want to show what role lifestyle has to play in strengthening the immune system and slowing and preventing inflammation in the body. Follow this advice and you will feel healthier and younger. It might also lead you to avoid a number of diseases and slow the biological ageing process.

I hope to be able to show you how your lifestyle can strengthen your own inherent powers. The healthier your habits, the more years of good health you can hope to enjoy. Let us begin with one of the most critical tips – the importance of movement.

TIP 1

● ●

Movement
rejuvenates the body

• • • • • • • • • • • • • • • • • • • •

We are designed to move about, so keeping the body active has a wide range of positive effects. In fact, some form of physical activity can cut the risk of around thirty to forty diseases including several types of cancer, cardiovascular diseases and diabetes. And yet some people still think they have no time for exercise.

If you don't set aside time for exercise today, you'll need to set aside even more time later in life – for being ill.

Exercise not only extends life, it also gives us more energy so we feel several years younger. People who begin to exercise or take moderate physical activity age more slowly than those who are inactive. A sixty-year-old can have the body of a forty-year-old, but on the other hand a forty-year-old can also have the body of a sixty-year-old.

No matter how old you are, or what physical condition you are in, exercise will always make the body younger.

But remember that this effect only lasts as long as you continue to exercise. Exercise is a perishable item, it can't be stored in the body, but has to be repeated on a regular basis.

HOW CAN PHYSICAL ACTIVITY MAKE THE BODY YOUNGER?

Physical activity affects the whole body, including the heart and blood vessels, the immune system, muscles, bones and mental well-being. To build up your body, you also need to eat well. What happens is that cells are repaired, new blood vessels form for increased blood flow, heart and lung capacity rises, and stress hormone levels fall, which leads to less inflammation and a stronger immune system.

Positive effects of physical exercise include:

Extended life expectancy

Generally speaking, physical activity leads to a longer life. Several studies have shown that regular physical activity can extend life by as much as eight years. Research has also shown a more than 50 per cent reduction in mortality among fit and active people compared with sedentary people.

Reduces stress

Regular physical activity reduces the symptoms of stress, which makes you feel more relaxed, healthier and better able to deal with life. This in turn reduces inflammation in the body and stems the ageing process.

Combats dementia

Research has shown that exercise causes a significant delay in the development of dementia. Physical activity improves long-term memory and slows ageing in the blood vessels.

Combats diabetes

Physical exercise strongly counteracts the risk factors behind diabetes-related illness and premature death.

Combats cancer

Physical exercise protects against certain forms of cancer, including breast cancer, prostate cancer, uterine cancer and bowel cancer.

Combats cardiovascular disease

Studies have shown that men who exercise are at half the risk of suffering a heart attack compared with those who do not exercise. Women who go walking are almost 50 per cent less likely to have a stroke than those who don't walk. People who have an active everyday life have a 30 per cent lower risk of suffering cardiovascular disease or premature death than people who have a sedentary life.

THREE TYPES OF GOOD PHYSICAL ACTIVITY

Any activity is a good activity, as long as it is fun, your own choice and easy to do, because then there is a better chance that you'll keep it up. The important and difficult thing is to get started and stay motivated. But by thinking about the positive effects of physical activity – reduced stress hormones, stronger immune defences, improved self-esteem, greater vitality, sharper mind, better sleep, improved productivity and happiness and a younger body – you may begin to look forward to your walk, bike ride or session at the gym!

To get as much as possible from your exercise, you need to remember that there are three basic types of physical activity: general, cardio exercise, and strength and flexibility exercises. They all affect the ageing process in different ways. Try to incorporate all three activities in your exercise plan.

General physical activity

This means everyday exercise. It has a good effect and there are opportunities to do it all the time, if you think about it. Walking, gardening, window cleaning, shopping, taking the stairs instead of the lift, leaving the car at home and going on foot or cycling instead – it all promotes good health and researchers increasingly stress the importance of everyday exercise. Just upping the level of general activity – without even breaking a sweat – can deliver 40 per cent of the rejuvenating effect that physical activity brings.

Cardio exercise

This means activities that get the heart beating faster, making you short of breath and preferably also a little sweaty. Examples of this include brisk walking and pole walking. If you choose to go jogging, a good rule of thumb is that the intensity should still allow you to talk to your running mate as you jog, but if you can sing the pace is too slow.

You can also get a good amount of exercise from activities such as dancing, badminton, tennis, football, skiing, skating, cycling, swimming and water aerobics. It is difficult to single out one specific kind of activity that is better than the others so choose the activity that suits you best. This type of exercise contributes a further 40 per cent to the rejuvenation that can be associated with physical activity.

Strength and flexibility exercises

After the age of thirty, your muscle mass slowly starts to reduce and this has to be counteracted in good time. Every percentage increase in muscle mass can add a year to your life. Building up and strengthening your muscles with weight training and then keeping them in shape can contribute 20 per cent to the overall reduction in ageing that comes from exercise. And this is an important 20 per cent, because strengthening the muscles and skeleton reduces the risk of muscle strains and joint injuries as you do the other types of physical activity.

HOW MUCH SHOULD YOU EXERCISE?

Little and often is the key – thirty minutes of 'everyday exercise' daily, according to the research. You can achieve additional health benefits by adding twenty to thirty minutes of running or equivalent activity three times a week.

Alternatively, you can combine these activities. Muscle-building physical activity is recommended at least twice a week for the majority of the body's major muscle groups.

Children and adolescents up to age eighteen are recommended to have sixty minutes of physical activity per day.

● ●

Research shows

A person who exercises for at least three hours a week is biologically ten years younger than someone who doesn't exercise.

● ●

Can you have too much exercise?

The advice is not to over-exercise. Research has shown that extreme training has no additional health benefits, but instead increases the risk of injury, including stress fractures. Marathon runners can suffer heart problems in the form of irregular heart rhythm, known as atrial fibrillation, as well as wear and tear to the hips and knees. In other words, as in so many things, moderation is the key.

Use a pedometer

You may find it stimulating to use a pedometer to see whether you're reaching the target you set yourself. Aim for 10,000—12,000 steps over the course of a whole day, which is equivalent to walking six to eight kilometres or four or five miles. Less than 5,000 steps is considered a 'sedentary lifestyle'.

ENERGY USE IN THIRTY MINUTES

If you use physical activity to keep control of your weight, it can be interesting for you to see which activities burn more or fewer calories. The figures in the table below are only approximate values for energy use as they vary depending on how much you weigh and how you define 'average' activity levels.

Common activities and their energy use per 30 minutes	
Gardening	150 kcal
Walking	150 kcal
Skating	250 kcal
Swimming	350 kcal
Skiing	350 kcal
Jogging/running	350 kcal

Table 1

CAN PHYSICAL ACTIVITY COMPENSATE FOR AN OTHERWISE SEDENTARY LIFE?

The problem of sitting still is on the rise. TV, smart phones and computers are stealing more and more time. Some people are inactive for 90 per cent of their waking hours. Such a sedentary daily lifestyle has proven a serious risk factor for many of the most common diseases.

Sitting still means that our large muscle groups, particularly the buttock and leg muscles, are not used, which can lead to poor blood circulation and a reduced metabolism. This in turn leads to a rise in blood sugar levels, which causes inflammation and raises the risk of cardiovascular disease, diabetes, cancer and premature death.

The health benefits of being active three times a week are thus heavily outweighed by an otherwise sedentary life.

Generally speaking, we have previously been focused on physical activity, but we are only now beginning to understand the importance of also avoiding a sedentary life.

• •

Research shows

Several major studies have indicated that sitting too much (particularly with no activity at all) increases the risk of diabetes and of suffering and dying from cardiovascular disease and cancer. This has proven to be the case even with vigorous training in your spare time!

In an experiment, young healthy men were instructed to be as physically inactive as they could for a period of two weeks. In just this short time, blood sugar levels were affected, fitness levels dropped and their blood lipid (fat) count rose. This in turn increased the risk of conditions such as diabetes and cardiovascular disease.

On the ends of the chromosomes sit 'telomeres', which affect how we and our cells age. Studies have shown that sitting still causes the telomeres to shorten, which means a shorter life compared with people who are more active.

● ●

Break up your time when sitting still

To avoid the issues caused by sitting still, avoid sitting for more than thirty to forty-five minutes at a time. Stand up and move about, go and get a coffee, talk to your work colleagues, or do something else. Just stretching your legs for a few minutes is enough to counter the negative effects of sitting still.

STAND UP FOR YOUR HEALTH

Standing up at work has been a huge health trend in Sweden over the last couple of years. The knowledge that it reduces the risk of all sorts of lifestyle diseases means that more and more people are choosing to work standing up.

Many now have height adjustable desks, so they can work standing up if they want to. Switching between standing and sitting makes the body feel better. Adopting a standing position reduces the amount of harmful blood lipids (fats), cuts the blood sugar level and reduces inflammation. This creates better conditions for a healthier heart and blood vessels. Shifting your weight from one leg to the other also stimulates the circulation.

Standing up to work activates the body and increases the rate at which you burn energy. So if you stood for two hours more a day, you could reduce your weight by up to ten kilos in one year.

TIP 2

. . . .

Time for recovery

• • • • • • • • • • • • • • • • • • • •

It has been scientifically proven that a less stressful existence improves health. So relax your shoulders and accept that:

Life is not just about surviving, it's about thriving.

The stress response has been vital for our survival and as such is essentially a positive function. The body prepares itself for fight or flight. But in modern society, we rarely need to physically fight to survive. However, the stress response is also triggered by mental tension, for example when you get angry, struggle with money or a boring job, or have too much to do.

Stress doesn't have to be caused by real threats either. You get the same experience of stress simply by imagining a threat or a difficult situation that doesn't actually exist and that might never happen. The body still reacts with a stress response. As such, you can sustain your stress, no matter how good life actually is, by regularly thinking about accidents that could happen to yourself or your family, potential illnesses or similarly disturbing scenarios. News on TV and in the press constantly feeds the development of new anxieties and stresses.

We now know that stress is just as harmful as smoking. But stress is a natural part of life and people can tolerate considerable levels of short-term stress. However, in today's society, where so many people are forever connected via email, smartphone and social media, there are enormous information flows to deal with and many decisions to make. Demands are tough in working life, the pace is fast and stress is expanding and becoming increasingly prolonged. If you don't take time to recover, your health can be seriously damaged.

DIFFERENT TYPES OF STRESS

Situations that cause stress may not always be negative. It could, for instance, be something big and important, and the stress response can then give you the extra energy you need to complete the task.

Stress can also be perceived differently from person to person and attitudes can vary when faced with the same situation. What one person sees as stressful, another might see as challenging or exciting. Different attitudes mean that some people sink into chronic stress of varying degrees, while others don't see a problem and so don't feel stressed at all.

Many find demands from other people tough to deal with, but sometimes the demands you place on yourself can bring the most stress. If you set the bar high and want everything to be perfect, that creates stress. If your self-worth is based on how you perform, it is easy to push yourself to extremes in order to feel that you are good enough. The key is to realise that your worth has nothing to do with your performance.

In certain situations, you can also become stressed by not having enough meaningful tasks or challenges in your life. Involuntary solitude, unemployment or a lack of goals and meaning in life can create hopelessness and feelings of stress.

WHAT HAPPENS IN THE BODY

Stress affects the whole body, eating up energy and consuming nutrients, draining the body's reserves. Stress hormones such as adrenaline and cortisol are released and they make blood pressure, blood sugar and blood lipid (fat) levels rise. This increases free radicals, inflammation in the body rises and the immune system is damaged, causing an increased risk of cardiovascular disease, diabetes, infection and cancer. Brief periods of stress are thought not to cause damage. The harm comes with long-term or repeated stress, perhaps for weeks, months and years.

● ●

Research shows

A Swedish study has concluded that people who suffer stress and hopelessness in middle age run a two to three times greater risk of later developing dementia.

A different study showed that stressed women run a three to five times greater risk of developing breast cancer than unstressed women.

● ●

Some people get stressed very easily. They get angry and impatient in traffic queues, shout at motorists who overtake them and blow up at the smallest of injustices. These people are at much greater risk of cardiovascular disease, in the form of stroke and heart attack.

FIND STRATEGIES TO COMBAT YOUR STRESS

Everyday exercise

One of the best means of recovery is to get active. When stressed, it is easy to drop physical activity to save time, but looking after your body and being as active as possible is actually particularly beneficial during such periods. Exercise is good because stress raises levels of stress hormones, while exercise breaks them down. The body releases a calming hormone, oxytocin, which gives a lovely sense of relaxation.

Sleep reinvigorates

Sleep is needed for the body and brain to recover and recharge. If you cut back on sleep because you 'don't have time', you will quickly lose energy and effectiveness. You will be worse at problem solving and you will find it more difficult to say no. In other words, you won't be able to fight the stress around you and instead you risk being drawn into it and becoming part of it.

Breathe properly

Breathing calmly and methodically is perhaps humankind's most effective anti-stress tool. Taking slow, deep breaths, right down to the stomach, gives the body and mind an opportunity to regroup and re-energise. Such breathing helps you to balance your inner demands concerning performance and provide space for recovery. Deep breathing increases the circulation and lowers the heart rate, reduces anxiety and strengthens the immune system but, above all, deep breathing creates a sense of well-being and an inner calm.

Learn to forgive

You can't change the past and if you have made a mistake, what's done is done. Stop fretting, start forgiving yourself and instead think: what did I learn from this? Then start afresh. It is also important to be able to accept an apology from others, forgive an injustice and then simply let go of the problem.

*Learning to forgive yourself
and others reduces anxiety, tension
and thus harmful stress.*

Regular recovery

Relaxation through meditation, yoga and mental training can effectively reduce feelings of stress. Many people find going out into the countryside or taking a walk has a calming effect. Massage has also been shown to release oxytocin, which reduces feelings of stress. Mindfulness is about consciously living in the moment and not letting your thoughts drift off into stressful planning or anxiety for the future.

Give yourself days when you can 'just be'. Meet up with friends, laugh and have fun. Spend time with pets. Read books, listen to music or play an instrument, sing in a choir – all this can break the stress pattern and allow you to wind down.

Take control

Demanding situations over which you have little control and that you aren't sure how to handle are stressful. Taking control of your situation is an important aspect of combating your stress. There is no time to do everything, so you need to focus on what is important. The key is to find a way to sort through or reduce the number of balls you have in the air.

Write a list of what is stressing you and what needs to be done. This gives you an overall picture and makes it easier to focus on what needs to be prioritised. Then cross off everything that has been done. Seeing the number of points shrink and knowing that you have achieved something gives a feeling of satisfaction. And that in turn reduces the stress.

Time out

Being reachable at all times, commenting on Facebook and answering emails can take up time that isn't there. So make yourself unreachable, decide whether and when you want to have contact with the world – focus instead and plan what you know has to be done.

Lower the bar – think 'good enough'

If people are asking too much of you, it is important to take up the problem with those concerned. The person in question may not have understood how bad their demands are making you feel and they may be open to a discussion that could lead to change.

If you are the one who has set the bar too high, you need to be self-critical and rethink. Try to see that you would feel so much better if you lowered the bar and became less stressed and irritated. Everyone around you will probably be pleased to see you happier and calmer. Doing everything perfectly comes with far too high a price.

Think 'good enough' – it makes your life easier, cuts stress and enables you to live a longer and happier life.

TIP 3

. . . .

Sleep fortifies

. . . .

Sleeping well is vital in maintaining good health. A good night's sleep greatly improves our well-being and our capacity to perform well the next day. Sleep leaves us feeling rested and makes it easier for us to concentrate and learn new things. Now scientists are beginning to realise just how important sleep is for health over the longer term, and sleep has proven to be a key lifestyle factor. Getting enough sleep can reduce the risk of a whole host of diseases.

WHAT HAPPENS DURING SLEEP?

Sleep is our most important source of recovery, giving the body an opportunity to regain its balance after a day of exertion. When we are active during the day, we consume energy and that puts a kind of 'wear' on the body. During sleep our batteries recharge and repairs are made, but these are very much dependent on us getting enough sleep.

Our heart rate, blood pressure, breathing rate and body temperature drop. Stress levels fall and the number of free radicals drops, which also causes inflammation in the body to reduce. At the same time, the immune system is built up and reinforced, as the body prepares for a new day of action.

• •

Research shows

Sleep supports a strong immune system, which reduces the risk of issues such as cardiovascular disease, diabetes, depression and chronic fatigue syndrome. Good sleep extends our life.

• •

WHAT COUNTS AS ENOUGH SLEEP?

Eight hours of sleep was long considered the ideal. Around ten years ago, however, a major American study showed that:

The optimal period of sleep is seven hours on average.

One surprising finding was that too little sleep and too much sleep were both associated with health risks. The risk of premature death was just as great for those who slept eight hours or more as it was for those who slept six hours or less per night.

A Swedish study of 70,000 women showed that both short sleepers and long sleepers ran a greater risk of premature death, particularly if they were physically inactive. Physically active long sleepers, however, had no higher mortality rate than those who slept seven hours a night. In other words, the negative effects of too much sleep were mitigated by physical activity.

Age is a factor that has to be taken into account with regard to the need for sleep. The need for sleep reduces throughout life and is thus greatest in children and young adults. A twenty-year-old might need over eight hours sleep, but by the age of sixty they may well be fine on little more than six hours.

TAKE A NAP

A study of 24,000 people showed that people who regularly slept in the afternoon ran an almost 40 per cent lower risk of suffering cardiovascular disease that led to death. It is, however, a good idea to take your nap (about twenty minutes seems to be the optimum length) in the middle of the day so as not to interfere with your night-time sleep.

TIPS FOR GOOD SLEEP

Sleep routine

Create a clear sleep routine. Try to go to bed and wake up at the same time every day. This will support your biological clock and strengthen your body.

Daylight

Spend time out in daylight, preferably in the morning. This reduces production of the sleep hormone melatonin and puts the body back on its daytime setting, ready for activity. This strengthens the biological clock and means that the evening darkness will then produce a new batch of the sleep hormone.

Exercise

Exercise releases stress-reducing endorphins, which make it easier to sleep at night and improve the quality of that sleep. Exercise should, however, be avoided immediately before going to bed.

Wind down

Begin winding down in the evening well before bedtime. Stop looking at your computer and phone. Try to put aside anything that might stress you. Write down things you need to remember for the next day. This makes it easier to stop thinking about what needs doing. Calming activities are good, such as reading a (not too exciting) book. Practise the art of relaxing before going to bed. Make bed a work-free zone.

Good sleeping environment

Air your bedroom and then lie on a comfortable bed in a quiet, cool and dark room. Darkness signals to the brain that it is night and stimulates the release of the sleep hormone melatonin.

Be careful with caffeine and alcohol

Caffeine and alcohol can disrupt sleep. Caffeine has a half-life in the body of six to eight hours. This means that if you drink two cups of coffee in the afternoon, caffeine equivalent to one cup of coffee will still be affecting your body by the evening. This can be enough to impair your ability to sleep. Alcohol might help you fall asleep, but it is terrible for helping you stay asleep. Metabolising alcohol creates stresses in the body, which cause you to wake intermittently, resulting in poor quality sleep.

Snoring – a warning sign

Around 10 per cent of those who regularly snore also suffer from sleep apnoea when asleep. This entails a total constriction of the airways for a brief moment. Breathing may be interrupted for anything from a few seconds to as much as a minute.

Snoring, and particularly sleep apnoea, leads to poor-quality sleep, which also has a negative impact on quality of life. It will make you feel abnormally tired during the day and you might find yourself having lapses of memory and concentration.

Sleep apnoea may be associated with a number of serious illnesses. The lower oxygen level in the blood forces the heart to work harder, while stress hormones and blood pressure increase. Without treatment, the damaging effects build up and, over the long term, can lead to a number of serious medical conditions, including cardiovascular disease, stroke, high blood pressure, diabetes and asthn... In addition, a person with sleep apnoea runs a six to seven times higher risk of being in a car accident due to tiredness.

TOP TIPS

- Try to sleep on your stomach or side.

- Try breathing aids that expand the airways (nasal strips and plastic dilators).

- If you have a cold, try a nasal spray.

- Avoid alcohol, tobacco and sleeping pills.

- If overweight, try shedding some of that weight.

TIP 4

· ·

Sun – but not too much

SUN AND VITAMIN D

When out in the sun, you are exposed to the sun's ultraviolet rays, UVA and UVB. It is the UVB rays that form the body's vitamin D when the skin cells are exposed to direct sunlight.

The sun is the best source of vitamin D. In addition to the sun, we obtain some vitamin D via our food, such as oily fish (salmon, herring, mackerel, eel), eggs and vitamin D enriched milk. It is interesting to note that a brief moment of sunbathing in the summer provides as much vitamin D as fifty glasses of milk!

In a Nordic winter and many cold climate countries, practically no vitamin D is formed via the sun and then food becomes the key. There is a risk of vitamin D deficiency and many diseases, including cancer and MS, have been found to be more frequent in less sunny countries.

What does vitamin D do?

Vitamin D could be described as a miracle molecule that is needed to keep many bodily functions working. Vitamin D is good for the nervous system and for skeletal health as it combats brittle bones (osteoporosis). It also regulates the hormone balance and improves the absorption of minerals and other vital nutrients from the gut. In addition, vitamin D activates and boosts the immune system and helps to inhibit inflammation, protecting us against a long list of diseases, including:

- Various cancers
- MS
- Diabetes
- Rheumatoid arthritis
- Depression
- Psoriasis
- Osteoporosis
- Infections
- Dementia
- Blood clots in the leg

Research shows

A study in southern Sweden followed 29,000 women for twenty years and then compared their sun habits, the incidence of various diseases and mortality. The study showed that the women who had most avoided the sun developed diabetes and blood clots, which led to twice the mortality over twenty years compared with those who sunbathed. Avoiding the sun was judged to be as great a risk factor as smoking, inactivity and being overweight when it came to cardiovascular disease and death.

In another study, researchers from centres such as the Karolinska Institutet in Sweden analysed data from over four million patients in thirteen countries. The countries were split into sunny countries – such as Spain, Australia, Singapore – and non-sunny, e.g. Sweden and other Nordic countries. The conclusion was that people from sunny countries run much less of a risk of many cancers, including cancer of the stomach, rectum, kidneys and bladder, prostate, breast and lungs. The reduction in risk averaged out at a little over 50 per cent. The likely reason for this remarkable result is thought to be that the sun stimulates the body's production of vitamin D.

VITAMIN D FROM SUNBATHING

A suntan is tempting and many view a tan as one of the main goals of the summer. But it doesn't take much UV radiation for the body to get enough vitamin D.

In a British summer, for example, getting some sun on your face and arms for a short time in the middle of the day is enough to cover your daily need of vitamin D. Nearer the equator, where the UV radiation is stronger, an even shorter time in the sun is needed. In other words, we don't need to bake in order for our body to have enough. Instead it just increases the risk of wrinkles and, in the worst case, skin cancer. More sun doesn't mean more vitamin D, as the skin shuts down production once levels have been topped up.

VITAMIN D FROM DIETARY SUPPLEMENTS

Since UVB radiation is filtered out by the atmosphere when the sun is low, in practice we only have the warmer half of the year, April/May to August/September, to produce vitamin D in decent quantities. This means that those of us who live at more northerly latitudes can't form vitamin D naturally with the sun's help in winter.

Vitamin D deficiency can shorten life, and it is one of the few vitamins that we risk getting too little of. An extra supplement of vitamin D in the winter can therefore be good for your health. There is no risk of toxicity if you keep to the recommended dose. High doses over long periods can, however, have toxic effects.

The NHS and the Swedish National Food Agency recommends a daily intake of 10 micrograms/400 IE, (IE=international units) for children and adults. Older people over seventy-five are recommended to take a double dose, 20 micrograms/800 IE per day. The vitamin D that you make from the sun in the summer can be stored for a few weeks into the autumn, but it gradually becomes depleted. It is therefore appropriate to start taking vitamin supplements at the autumnal equinox and stop at the spring equinox.

SUN ADVICE

Get some sun daily during the summer. The sun is in short supply in northern latitudes, so stock up with vitamin D. You don't have to lie on a beach in swimwear to get some sun. The sun has its beneficial vitamin D effect just as much on someone working in the garden, taking a walk or lying in a hammock in shorts and a T-shirt.

To make sure you get your important daily dose of vitamin D, you should sunbathe for fifteen to twenty minutes without sunscreen or a very low factor sunscreen. The sunscreen filters out UVB rays and so almost no vitamin D is formed. Sunbathe in the middle of the day, since the sun provides the most vitamin D when it is highest in the sky. If you work indoors all day, try to get outside at lunchtime: take a walk or have a coffee in the sun.

If you intend to stay in the sun longer than twenty minutes, sunscreen should be used and remember: don't get burnt. Avoid showering and using soap immediately after sunbathing, as the fat-soluble vitamin D will be washed away. It takes a few hours for it to be absorbed through the skin into the body.

Use sunglasses to protect your eyes from UV light and reduce the risk of cataracts.

A good way of boosting vitamin D in winter is, if possible, to take a holiday to a warmer climate.

SUNBATHING CAUSES MORE BENEFIT THAN HARM

Sunbathing boosts health and keeps many diseases at bay. Professor Edward Giovannucci of Harvard University reported back in 2005 that:

Thirty people die of diseases related to vitamin D deficiency for every one who dies of skin cancer.

But this is only true if you are careful with your sunbathing and don't burn. The risk of developing a malignant melanoma later in life is greater if you had sunburn as a child. If you are in a risk group for malignant melanoma, you should also be very careful about being exposed to the sun's rays. Risk factors include being blond, ginger or freckly, having many birthmarks or having skin cancer in your family history. If you are in such a group, you should protect yourself against the sun, preferably with clothing rather than sunscreen. Care should always be exercised when it comes to children's exposure to the sun.

TIP 5

· ·

Eat yourself healthy

• • • • • • • • • • • • • • • • • • •

Over the past fifteen years, hundreds of thousands of new studies have been published about diet. And yet there is still a great deal of uncertainty, with the advice continually changing. One reason for this is the difficulty in conducting and interpreting diet-related studies.

Yet, within this bulk of information, there are certain facts that researchers agree on. It is, for example, accepted that certain foods have clear links to health and to disease. 'You are what you eat' is proving increasingly true. The benefits of eating properly include a longer and healthier life.

FOOD CAN BOTH PROTECT AGAINST AND CREATE INFLAMMATION

In the introduction, I described how insidious inflammation damages the body, causing problems such as infection, cancer, cardiovascular disease, diabetes and dementia. Research has shown, in recent years, that a particular type of food causes serious inflammation in the body by increasing the quantity of free radicals.

There are also foods that strengthen our vital immune system and that protect against and even cure inflammation.

These are:

- Antioxidants

- Omega-3 and omega-6 in the right proportions

- Food with a low glycaemic index (GI)

- Fibre and probiotics

ANTIOXIDANTS

Food contains something called antioxidants. There are several substances that function as antioxidants, including vitamin A, vitamin B2 and B5, vitamin C, vitamin E, riboflavin and selenium. Copper, manganese and zinc also play an important role, not least because they are part of various compounds with an antioxidant effect. The different types of antioxidant work together as a team, so you need to consume all the types for them to have their full effect.

> *The body can produce its own antioxidants, but production falls away from the age of twenty-five. Antioxidants therefore need to be sourced via food and drink.*

Antioxidants take care of free radicals

Free radicals attack and damage the body's cells and functions, as well as contributing to ageing and various kinds of disease. The antioxidants serve as a security force that tracks down the free radicals formed in the body and neutralises them. As long as the security force is strong enough, the number of free radicals are kept to a low level in the body.

Antioxidants also protect against harmful genes

Another exciting discovery is that antioxidants can also determine whether a particular gene we are carrying will cause disease. We know that certain genes are linked to various diseases, including diabetes, Parkinson's, Alzheimer's and various forms of cancer. Few are aware that such genes may well not cause a problem as long as they are not activated.

Free radicals are a powerful activating factor, but if the protective antioxidants prevent the free radicals from attacking, the genes can remain passive and harmless.

Which foods contain antioxidants?

Fruit and berries are a rich source of antioxidants. Go for your preferred choice and vary that choice according to the season. Choose fruit and berries of different colours according to the rainbow method to get plenty of different antioxidants, see table 2.

Take note of the dozen types of fruit and vegetables (called the 'Dirty Twelve') which contain so much pesticide that they should only be consumed in organic form. They are labelled 'organic' in tables 2 and 3. (Potatoes are also among the Dirty Twelve, but they don't make it onto the list of the best antioxidants below.) If there is no organic option, buy a different, non-toxic kind of fruit or vegetable instead. Sometimes there is a frozen alternative, which is a good choice. Dried fruit is also an effective way to consume plenty of antioxidants.

Best list: fruit and berries			
apples (organic)	apricots	aronia berries	bananas
blackberries	blackcurrants	blueberries	cherries
cranberries	dates	goji berries	gooseberries
grapefruit	kiwi fruit	lemons	lingonberries
nectarines (organic)	oranges	peaches (organic)	pears
plums	pomegranates	prunes	raisins
raspberries	red grapes (organic)	sea buckthorn	strawberries (organic)

Table 2

When it comes to vegetables, eat lots of them in different colours and for every meal. Choose vegetables from the list of the best, with high levels of antioxidants, see table 3.

Best list: vegetables			
aubergine	avocado	beans	beetroot
broccoli	Brussels sprouts	carrot	cauliflower
celery (organic)	cucumber (organic)	garlic	green cabbage
iceberg lettuce	melon (organic)	onion	peas
rhubarb	red pepper (organic)	salad leaves	spinach (organic)
sugar snap peas	sweet potato	tomato (organic)	white cabbage

Table 3

How much fruit and veg should you eat?

Set yourself a target of eating fruit and vegetables for every meal. A suitable quantity per day is 500–700 grams (e.g. three to four items of fruit and two to three portions of vegetables). To keep a proper check on the weights, it can be worth using scales occasionally.

These figures are a challenge for most people, with only one-third of the British population eating the recommended amount, for example. Don't be afraid to try new berries, fruit and vegetables, fresh or frozen – shops carry a huge range nowadays.

Avoid heat

Most antioxidants are destroyed at temperatures between 30–100°C. Cooking in a microwave, for example, eliminates practically all the antioxidants. If possible, opt for gentle stir-frying or steaming. One exception is tomatoes, which need a certain amount of cooking to release their antioxidant (lycopene). Tomato sauce, tomato purée and tinned tomatoes are therefore particularly good.

Other sources of antioxidants

Many herbs and spices can be rich in antioxidants, see table below.

Best list: herbs and spices			
basil	black pepper	caraway	cardamom
cayenne pepper	chilli pepper	cinnamon	cloves
curry powder	dill	ginger	mint
mustard seeds	oregano	parsley	rosemary
sage	thyme	turmeric	

Table 4

Of the above herbs and spices, it is worth saying that turmeric has the strongest anti-inflammatory effect. Turmeric makes up 20 per cent of curry powder. In India, for example, people eat turmeric daily and suffer five to fifty times fewer cancer cases (depending on the type of cancer) compared with Westerners of the same age. It is not surprising then that turmeric has been dubbed Asian gold! Note, however, that turmeric can't be absorbed through the intestinal wall unless it is mixed with pepper or ginger. Turmeric should be avoided if pregnant and breast-feeding, and an overdose can cause a number of side effects.

• •

Super drink with turmeric (created by Professor Stig Bengmark)

1 tbsp turmeric

1 tsp cinnamon

¼ tsp chilli pepper

cayenne pepper or black pepper

1 tbsp lemon juice

1 tbsp apple cider vinegar

1 tbsp olive or coconut oil

Stir the spices into the lemon juice, apple cider vinegar and olive oil or coconut oil.

Mix in a glass with 100–200 ml blackcurrant juice (or oat milk, water – find your favourite), drink once a day. You can also try replacing the liquid with something like oatmeal mixed with apple purée or your favourite berries for a better flavour.

● ●

Nuts are also nutritious. They contain a range of anti-inflammatory substances and also facilitate the absorption of antioxidants. Nuts are very rich in energy and fat so should be consumed in moderation – approximately a handful of mixed nuts per day. Almonds are included in the table, but they are not actually nuts in a strictly botanical sense.

Best list: nuts				
almonds	cashews	hazelnuts	pecans	walnuts

Table 5

Look out for old walnuts, check to be sure they are not past their use-by date. Discoloured or mouldy nuts can contain the carcinogenic substance aflatoxin. Throw away the whole bag!

They can contain large quantities of trans fats, which can damage the vascular system. Walnuts are best kept in the fridge as they are sensitive to heat and sunlight.

Linseeds (flaxseeds) are really nutritious seeds that contain antioxidants and they can be mixed into breakfast cereals. Like other high-fibre foods they can, however, cause digestive problems in people with a sensitive gut. Eat no more than two tablespoons of linseeds per day as they can contain a small amount of toxic cyanide compounds.

Don't go overboard with pumpkin seeds, sunflower seeds and pine nuts due to their content of omega-6.

Finally, chocolate also contains antioxidants and the recommended type is dark chocolate with at least 70 per cent cocoa. Eat a few squares (not too many!) instead of biscuits with your coffee or tea. Some studies claim that any chocolate with cocoa has a positive health effect.

•••••••••••••••••••••••••••••••••••••

Research shows

Two recently published studies showed that high chocolate intake was linked with a lower risk of both cardiovascular disease and stroke. Surprisingly, the results came from eating all forms of chocolate! For the time being, however, the recommendation of 70 per cent cocoa remains in place.

•••••••••••••••••••••••••••••••••••••

OMEGA-3 AND OMEGA-6 IN THE RIGHT PROPORTIONS

Omega-3

Omega-3 is a healthy polyunsaturated fatty acid that humans are unable to produce for themselves. We therefore have to source it from our food. Found primarily in fish and shellfish, omega-3 increases the quantities of the hormone-like substances eicosanoids, which in turn have a powerful anti-inflammatory effect, see table 6.

Best list: fish and shellfish			
anchovies	herring	king crab	lobster
mackerel	mussels	prawns	rainbow trout
salmon	sardines	tuna	

Table 6

People who eat fish several times a week have a much lower risk of contracting many forms of cancer. Note that frozen fish loses some of its omega-3 content over time.

The NHS recommends two portions of fish or shellfish every week and no more than four portions of oily fish, unless pregnant or breastfeeding, in which case do not exceed more than two portions. You should avoid eating wild-caught fish, since they can often contain high levels of environmental toxins (mercury, PCB, dioxin). The question of whether farmed salmon should be recommended is currently under discussion.

Omega-3 can also be found in oils, seeds, nuts and vegetables, see table 7 for the best list.

Best list: oils, seeds, nuts and vegetables			
avocado	chia seeds	coconut oil	cod liver oil
green cabbage	linseeds (flaxseeds)	linseed (flaxseed) oil	olives
olive oil	rapeseed oil	spinach	walnuts

Table 7

Meat and dairy products can contain good quantities of omega-3, as long as the animals have been reared outdoors and grazed on fresh grass. Eggs are also a good source of omega-3, but they should come from free range hens.

• •

Research shows

A major Swedish study showed that unsaturated fats in olive and rapeseed oils cut the risk of breast cancer by almost 50 per cent. All it took to achieve this effect was to replace a tablespoon of fat (margarine) with olive or rapeseed oil.

• •

Omega-6

Omega-6 (linoleic acid) is important for our immune system and is a healthy polyunsaturated fatty acid if consumed in the right quantity. We are unable to produce it ourselves, so it has to be sourced from our food. Prehistoric humans consumed more or less equal amounts of omega-3 and omega-6, which had positive health effects. As humanity has evolved, however, our eating habits have changed considerably and now our diet may contain twenty times more omega-6 than omega-3 and, in this ratio, omega-6 has an inflammatory effect.

Researchers believe this imbalance in our intake of fatty acids is a strong contributor to the increase in inflammation and impaired immune defences

Note that the 'organic' label means a product contains no pesticides, hormones or antibiotics. It may, however, still be high in omega-6 and low in omega-3, so look out for the labels 'grass-fed' or 'rich in omega-3'.

There are foods rich in omega-6 that should be cut down, see table 8, below.

Foods to cut down
• biscuits, cakes, sweets, white bread
• corn oil, sunflower oil, soya oil, palm oil
• eggs from non-free-range hens
• hydrogenated fats (trans fats), margarine
• mayonnaise, bottled dressing
• meat from non-grass-fed animals
• roasted onion, fries, crisps
• sunflower seeds, sesame seeds, pumpkin seeds, pine nuts

Table 8

CHOOSE FOOD WITH A LOW RATHER THAN HIGH GLYCAEMIC INDEX

The body needs carbohydrates for energy. However, there are slow-release and fast-release carbohydrates. The glycaemic index (GI) is a measure of how fast blood sugar levels rise after a meal (see figure 3 on page 76).

Eating food with a low glycaemic index, which means slow carbohydrates (see table 9), leads to a low/moderate rise in blood sugar levels and insulin, which in turn keeps inflammation in the body at low levels.

Food and drink that releases energy quickly – fast carbohydrates (see table 10, page 78) – has a high GI. This means blood sugar levels rise rapidly, as do insulin levels, increasing the degree of inflammation. Food with a high GI thus increases the risk of cancer, contributes to arteriosclerosis and cardiovascular diseases and is linked with the development of diabetes and dementia.

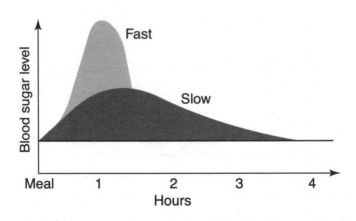

Figure 3. Fast carbohydrates (high GI) cause a spike in blood sugar levels. Slow carbohydrates (low GI) give a gentle/moderate rise in blood sugar levels

Best list: low GI
• apples
• apricots
• bananas (unripe)
• beans such as kidney, soya, haricot
• berries such as blackberries, blueberries, lingonberries, raspberries, strawberries
• breads such as multigrain, sourdough
• brown rice
• cereals such as bran, bran flakes, natural muesli
• cherries
• chocolate, dark 70 per cent
• grapefruit
• grapes
• lemons
• lentils
• nuts such as almonds, peanuts
• oatmeal
• onions
• oranges
• peaches
• pears
• peas
• plums
• wholegrain pasta
• yoghurt, natural

Table 9. Food and drink with slow carbohydrates

Don't worry too much if you can't find specific GI values for individual foods. The figures will vary anyway depending on how the foods are prepared. What counts is the total GI of the whole meal.

Worst list: high GI
• bananas (yellow)
• beer, sweet wine
• biscuits, cakes, wafers, waffles
• breads such as baguettes, burger buns, croissants, flatbread, gluten-free, non-wholegrain crispbreads, pittas, toast, teacakes, white bread
• cereals such as cornflakes, oat crisp, puffed rice, sugar puffs
• couscous
• easy cook rice
• honey
• ice cream, sorbet
• jam, marmalade
• liquorice
• baked potato, French fries, mashed potato, potato sticks
• soda, energy drinks, juice, sports drinks
• syrup, sugar, brown sugar
• sweets
• wheat bread, rice cakes

Table 10. Food and drink with fast carbohydrates

FIBRE AND PROBIOTICS

Fibre is a carbohydrate that can't be broken down in the small intestine and therefore reaches the large intestine mostly unchanged. Some fibre stimulates bowel movements and makes food digestion more efficient. Other types of fibre contribute to a more even blood sugar level and lower fat content in the blood.

We have an incredible number of useful bacteria in our gut that extract vital nutrients from food and transfer them to the body to keep it fit and healthy. Eating a bacteria-friendly diet that is rich in fibre (see table 11) can also keep our precious bacteria working in optimum partnership with our immune system.

Fibre

Most Westerners eat less than half the recommended amount of fibre (e.g. three slices of wholegrain bread per day) which puts us at greater risk of falling ill. Increasing our fibre intake would boost our health.

Research shows

A study in the US monitored 75,000 women over a period of ten years and found that eating fibre-rich wholegrain products reduced the risk of cardiovascular disease.

Higher consumption of fibre can also reduce the risk of diabetes, intestinal and bowel cancer and breast cancer, and lead to a longer life.

Best list: high-fibre food			
Wholegrain products			
bulgur wheat	millet	natural muesli	quinoa
rye flakes	wheat germ	wholegrain bread	wholegrain cereals
wholegrain pasta	wholegrain porridge oats	wholegrain rice	
Fruit, vegetables, seeds			
artichoke	asparagus	banana (unripe or green)	beans
brassicas	carrot	garlic	leek
lentils	linseeds (flaxseeds)	peas	red onion

Table 11

Many high-fibre products can be eaten in large quantities, but some should be eaten in moderation. The problem is that they can cause a build-up of gas, stomach swelling and pain. People vary greatly in their reaction to different fibre products, so it is worth finding what works for you.

Probiotics

The daily consumption of probiotics, which are beneficial bacteria (lacto, acidofilus and bifido bacteria), is also good for your gut flora. Harmful bacteria can release endotoxins that cause inflammation if they enter the body. Fibre and probiotics protect against this, therefore inhibiting the development of chronic diseases and extending our lives.

Probiotics can be found in acidic foods that have been fermented through exposure to bacteria and yeasts without air access, such as sauerkraut, sour milk and yoghurt, but also in onions, tomatoes and so on.

OTHER DIETARY ADVICE

Meat is an important source of protein – but choose wisely

Meat provides protein and many nutrients and is also an important source of iron. Research has, however, shown that red meat (which includes beef, pork and lamb) increases the risk of cancer in the large intestine and bowel. The risk is even greater when it comes to processed meat products. The research has not yet pinpointed what in red meat and processed meats is behind the increased risk of these cancers. There may be several factors that interact. Those under consideration include fat, nitrites, nitrosamines, salt, viruses and the form of iron found in meat.

Good choices are:

- Chicken, turkey and other poultry

- Game

- Beef from grass-fed cows

Limit consumption

The current advice is to limit consumption of red meat to three normal-sized portions a week. You should also restrict your intake of processed meats. These are meat products that have been treated with nitrites, smoked or cured in some other way. Examples include sausage, bacon, salami, smoked ham, pâté and black pudding.

The Department of Health in the UK and the Swedish National Food Agency recommends eating no more than 500 grams of red meat and processed meats per week, and processed meats should account for only a small proportion of that amount.

Avoid industrially manufactured trans fats

Researchers agree on the harmful effects of hydrogenated and partially hydrogenated fats, so-called trans fats, which are industrially manufactured.

They have a negative effect on blood lipids (fats) and constitute a major risk factor for both cardiovascular disease and cancer.

Trans fats have one major practical advantage: they don't go rancid, and that is why they are used in many of the foods that can spend weeks and months on supermarket shelves. In other words, there are commercial motives for using these harmful trans fats. It is important to read the list of ingredients in order to avoid trans fats. Avoid any products where the fats are labelled as 'hydrogenated' or 'partially hydrogenated'. Hydrogenated fat may sometimes be disguised as 'vegetable fat'. A good strategy can be to choose products that specify the fats or that declare the product to be free from hydrogenated fats. Be careful with imported cakes and biscuits, which can contain relatively high levels of trans fats.

Be careful with purchased food such as cakes, biscuits, buns, wafers, mayonnaise, ice cream, pies, pasties, pizza, crisps and deep-fried food such as French fries.

Research shows

Denmark introduced restrictions on industrially
manufactured trans fats in food, and this was followed
by a greater reduction in mortality from cardiovascular
disease than in any other country during the same
period.

Natural trans fats

Trans fats occur naturally in produce such as nuts (look out
for old walnuts), dairy products and meat from cows and
sheep. There is a debate about whether natural trans fats
are as harmful as the industrially produced trans fats – the
Swedish National Food Agency maintains that they are,
but many researchers disagree.

Saturated fat – good or bad?

Saturated fat can be found in products such as chocolate,
baked goods, ice cream, full fat milk, butter and spreads
based on butter, palm oil, coconut oil, cheese, fat, meat and
processed meats such as sausage and bacon.

Eating saturated fats has long been considered harmful. But the risk in advising low consumption of saturated fats is that we instead replace them with fast carbohydrates. This causes high insulin levels and constantly elevated blood sugar levels, which in turn cause widespread inflammation in our body and hasten the ageing process. We need instead to increase our consumption of the healthy fats and oils to make us feel full and healthy.

Recent studies show that saturated fat may not be as harmful as previously thought. Some researchers believe, for example, that butter is better for us than margarine.

When it comes to milk and dairy products, the recommendations from researchers also vary. Several studies indicate, however, that soured products such as yoghurt and sour milk are preferable to regular milk due to the presence of healthy bacteria and less lactose.

TO SUM IT UP

Eat plenty of the healthy stuff and you'll be okay with the rest.

This tip comes from Peter Nilsson, professor of cardiovascular research at the University of Lund, in Sweden. The main thrust of his advice is that if you eat vegetables with every meal, you will be consuming antioxidants that can protect you against the free radicals formed from the rest of your diet. This means that if you let your food choices slip a little on occasion, you can still reduce the risk of harm by also eating good food at the same time.

The same is true if you eat food with a high GI. The harmful effects are reduced if at the same time you eat food with a low GI, as this brings down the overall GI value for the whole meal. If sugar is combined with other foods – particularly vegetables or nutritious fats – this delays the absorption of the sugar by the body, evening out the blood sugar and insulin peaks and reducing the level of inflammation.

TIP 6

· · · · · · · · · · · · · · · · · · · ·

Choose the right drink

• • • • • • • • • • • • • • • • • • • •

Food is by no means the only factor in achieving good
health and a longer life. Certain drinks can also help to
promote health. Of course water is the number one drink
for life. We can last countless days without food, but take
away water or other fluids and we can only last a few days
without complications occurring.

Drinking enough fluids creates a healthy environment for
the whole of our body. If we take in too little fluid every
day, the body will constantly be operating at a dehydrated
level, which can give rise to many symptoms and diseases.
Simply drinking much more fluid than we would normally
on a daily basis can help us to maintain better general
health. The recommended quantity of fluid per day is 1.5
litres

When it comes to other drinks, the main focus is on coffee,
tea and alcohol.

COFFEE

Finland and Sweden are the first and second biggest coffee drinking nations in the world. Coffee contains both caffeine and antioxidants and several studies show that coffee has a beneficial effect on health. Caffeine is a stimulant, while antioxidants strengthen the immune system and combat inflammation.

A cup of coffee contains 100–150 mg caffeine and the effect of one cup can last for several hours. This explains why some people can find it hard to sleep at night if they drink coffee too late in the afternoon.

There is plenty of scientific evidence that in moderate amounts, three to four cups a day, coffee has a beneficial effect on health. It can therefore be recommended, as long as you like coffee and it doesn't cause stomach problems or other side effects. But be careful about coffee-based drinks that contain large quantities of sugar and saturated fat (cream and milk). Coffee drinking can also be associated with the unhealthy consumption of biscuits and cakes.

Since research has shown that even decaffeinated coffee has health benefits, it is not entirely clear which substances in the coffee are actually good for your health. It is likely, however, that antioxidants (see page 62) account for the majority of the positive effect.

● ●

Research shows

Reduced risk of diabetes

A large US study which monitored 125,000 people over twenty years showed that increasing coffee consumption by one cup a day reduced the risk of diabetes, irrespective of what your coffee intake was from the start.

An even bigger study of around 450,000 people showed that those who drank three to four cups of coffee a day had a 25 per cent lower risk of developing diabetes than people who drank up to two cups of coffee a day.

Reduced risk of stroke

A study which monitored 80,000 women over the course of twenty years found that those who drank two to three cups of coffee a day ran an almost 20 per cent lower risk of suffering a stroke than women who rarely drank coffee. Interestingly, decaffeinated coffee also reduced the risk of a stroke, but to a lesser degree than ordinary coffee with caffeine.

Reduced risk of Alzheimer's

A Swedish-Finnish study showed that middle-aged people who drank three to five cups of coffee a day had around a 60 per cent lower risk of developing Alzheimer's compared with those who only drank up to two cups a day. The researchers believed the most likely explanation was that the coffee's high levels of antioxidants gave protection to the brain.

Reduced risk of Parkinson's disease

Studies have shown that caffeine can reduce the risk of developing Parkinson's disease. Those who drank three cups of coffee every day over a twenty-year period had only half the risk of developing Parkinson's.

Reduced risk of cancer recurrence

A study in Lund showed that women who drank more than two cups of coffee a day ran less of a risk of breast cancer recurrence. Another study found that coffee drinking was linked to fewer recurrences of bowel cancer.

• •

TEA

Like coffee, tea contains caffeine and has a generally stimulating effect. A cup of tea contains 40–50 mg, which is around half the level in coffee. This is the case for black, green and white tea. Rooibos (red bush tea) and herbal teas contain no caffeine.

Tea (black, green and white) is also rich in antioxidants, which combat inflammation and protect the immune system. Like coffee, tea has therefore been shown to reduce the risk of stroke, diabetes and cardiovascular disease. The amount of antioxidants in a cup of tea is similar to the amount in two apples or seven glasses of orange juice. Herbal tea, however, does not contain large amounts of antioxidants. Yerba mate tea is rich in antioxidants, but with less caffeine, and is considered to have its own positive health effects.

ALCOHOL

This is a sensitive subject, for so many reasons. Alcohol can be a help and a hindrance. Regular alcohol consumption in small quantities is thought to promote health and reduce the risk of various diseases. Too much alcohol, on the other hand, can lead to a litany of diseases and premature death.

Unfortunately, consumption is not evenly spread across the population, with around 10 per cent drinking 50 per cent of the alcohol consumed. It is this 10 per cent that have the biggest problems with alcohol.

So what is the right balance? Firstly, the positive health effects of alcohol consumption do not come until you reach the age when the risk of cardiovascular disease rises, which is in middle age. Alcohol has absolutely no positive effect on the health of younger people.

Secondly, the positive effect on health only applies to those who drink in moderation. It is therefore up to each of us to decide whether alcohol should be part of a health promoting lifestyle. Drinking to get drunk wipes out any positive effects from the alcohol and instead poses a risk of alcohol abuse, with all the major medical and social problems that this entails.

If a man and a woman drink the same amounts of alcohol, the woman will tend to have a higher blood alcohol level than the man. This is because when we drink alcohol it is diluted in the water contained in our body. Women, on average, weigh less than men and therefore have less body fluid. In addition, alcohol is broken down in the liver by the same system that breaks down the female hormone oestrogen, which means that the liver is slower at breaking down alcohol in women. These various factors are interdependent, which means that in some countries there are different limits for alcohol intake and high-risk consumption for men and women.

In the UK, high-risk consumption is considered to be consumption that exceeds fourteen units for men and women, which should be spread across three days or more.

To convert the strength of different alcoholic drinks to unit equivalents:

175 ml glass of wine = 2.1 units

250 ml glass of wine = 3 units

Pint of 5 per cent or above beer/cider = 3 units

Shot (25 ml) of spirit = 1 unit

Can red wine promote health?

Red wine contains many polyphenols, including the super-antioxidant resveratrol. It is formed in the grape's skin and seeds, which are incorporated into the fermentation process. White wine, where the skin is removed in the production process, therefore doesn't contain as many polyphenols. Resveratrol has a positive effect on genes that are known to protect healthy cells from ageing and can also impede cancer development. There are also other types of antioxidants in the wine, which reduce inflammation and thus protect the immune system. Even alcohol-free wine contains antioxidants. Pinot noir appears to have the very highest levels of resveratrol, but generally speaking the darker, more rustic and drier the wine, the more antioxidants it contains. So perhaps that explains why the French toast goes: *'à votre sant'* – 'to your health'!

•••••••••••••••••••••••••••••••

Research shows

Reduced risk of cardiovascular disease
Several major studies indicate that regular low to moderate intake of alcohol in middle and older age

significantly reduces the risk of developing or dying from cardiovascular disease.

A report by the Swedish Council on Health Technology Assessment (SBU) states that people with diabetes who regularly drink moderate amounts of alcohol run a lower risk of developing or dying from cardiovascular disease than those who do not drink alcohol.

Reduced risk of diabetes

According to a Finnish study that followed over 11,000 pairs of twins for twenty years, moderate consumption (such as one to two glasses of wine a day) reduced the risk of developing diabetes by 30 per cent for men and 40 per cent for women.

Reduced risk of rheumatoid diseases

A Scandinavian study has shown a 40–50 per cent reduction in the risk of rheumatoid diseases in those who drank alcohol regularly compared with those who didn't.

● ●

TO SUM IT UP

Drinking in moderation – preferably red wine – appears to have positive health effects from middle age onwards. However, reports are also coming out that question the benefits of alcohol. In other words, more research is needed to gain firmer answers.

Drinking alcohol on a daily basis can also be dubious advice, since even low to moderate intake may put some people at risk of developing a dependency. It is thus essential to remain vigilant about your relationship with alcohol.

If you are teetotal, you should not start drinking alcohol simply to reduce the risk of disease. Bearing in mind the downsides of alcohol, there are many less risky ways to promote health.

High-risk consumption and abuse are always harmful and contribute to a whole host of diseases, as well as premature death.

TIP 7

••••••••••••••••••••

Keep your weight in check

• • • • • • • • • • • • • • • • • • •

One health issue that affects many people but is quite
emotionally charged is weight gain. Over the years a huge
range of slimming books and newspaper articles about
different kinds of diets have been published. But despite
all the information about nutrition, diet and the health
problems associated with being overweight, the weight of
the general population just keeps rising.

Being overweight can cause many conditions that speed
up the body's ageing process. Being overweight and obese
are associated with increased inflammation, not least
because it causes a change in the bacterial flora of the gut,
which leads to more inflammatory endotoxins spreading
through the body. This in turn leads to conditions such
as high blood pressure, diabetes and cardiovascular
disease. Cancer is also more prevalent in people who are
overweight.

TRENDY DIETS ARE NO LONG-TERM SOLUTION

Most health authorities agree that there is no magic trick to dieting – all the fad diets eventually lead back to the starting weight. Constantly gaining and losing weight stresses the body and speeds up the ageing process.

Losing weight and then maintaining your ideal weight always involves switching to a lifestyle of healthy eating and exercise that is then maintained for life.

BUT WHAT IS NORMAL WEIGHT?

You don't need to battle to be slim, but not being overweight can add years to your life.

BMI

The most common way of calculating your weight is to determine your Body Mass Index (BMI), which takes account of the ratio between height and weight. (If you are very muscular, BMI is not an accurate measure.)

How to work out your BMI

Divide your body weight in kg by your height in metres squared.

Example: A person who weighs 70 kg and is 1.75 metres tall has a BMI of:

$$\frac{70}{1.75 \times 1.75} = 22.8$$

BMI for adults	
Underweight	Under 18.5
Normal weight	18.5–24.9
Overweight	25–29.9
Obese	30 or over

Abdominal fat

Harmful fat is the fat that gathers around the waistline. It is more harmful to be fat around the abdomen than it is to be heavy overall.

Research shows

Research has shown that abdominal fat is a different kind of fat than the type stored on the thighs, for example. The fat cells in the abdomen are active and when stressed, fatty acids are released into the blood, causing damage to the heart, arteries, liver and pancreas. Abdominal obesity also reduces the effectiveness of insulin and causes inflammatory substances to form. This leads to a greater risk of conditions such as cardiovascular disease, high blood pressure, stroke, diabetes and several forms of cancer.

●●●●●●●●●●●●●●●●●●●●●●●●●●●●●●●●●●●●●●●

How to measure your stomach

An easy way to quickly check your weight is to take a measuring tape and place it around your stomach. The measuring tape should run about two centimetres below the navel. Make sure the tape is horizontal and hasn't slid up your back. Breathe out gently when taking the measurement.

Figure for men	
Under 94 cm	healthy
Between 94 and 101	some health risk
Over 101	clear health risk

Figure for women	
Under 80 cm	healthy
Between 80 and 88	some health risk
Over 88	clear health risk

There is an increase in morbidity for every centimetre above the healthy value.

Stomach height

A new way of measuring this harmful abdominal fat (the fat that is embedded in and around the organs in the abdomen) is to lie down and measure the height of your stomach above the floor.

Lie on your back on the floor (or some other hard surface) with your knees bent so your back is in contact with the floor.

Place a ruler (or spirit level) horizontally over your stomach at navel height. Using another ruler, measure the height from the floor to the ruler on your stomach. Don't hold your breath, measure at the point of gently breathing out.

Healthy figure	
For men	under 22 cm
For women	under 20 cm

Keep your weight in check – a few general tips

It is all about:

- Eating and living well in a new way

- Not worrying about specialist diets or slimming cures

- Instead, remembering to eat nutritious, tasty food, regularly and in moderation – and then the weight loss will happen naturally

Don't leave the table stuffed

We have lost all control over the size of our food portions, which have doubled over the past twenty years. Muffins have become three times larger than they once were and burgers have also tripled in size. These big portions have encouraged us to eat more.

A good approach to food is not to eat until absolutely full. Start by not taking such large portions. Think two-thirds, so instead of three potatoes have two, and so on. It is no great sacrifice, but if you add this up over a month, it could mean as many as thirty to forty fewer potatoes. And that is good for your waistline! Cut up the pizza, two-thirds can be enough to give a good feeling of satisfaction, and share that giant pastry – it contains the same calories as an entire lunch!

Eat slowly – don't have seconds

Don't just think about what you eat, but also how you eat. If you bolt your food down, you won't have time to feel any sense of fullness and it will be very easy to have seconds because you'll still feel hungry. As well as causing weight gain, this will overload the digestive system, risking an upset stomach and indigestion. You will also be tired after this heavy meal.

If you eat slowly instead, chewing well and taking time to enjoy every mouthful, you'll notice when your stomach is full and when it is time to stop eating, as the fullness signals reach the brain. These take ten to fifteen minutes to occur, but if you wait for this feeling of fullness, it is easier to stop yourself from having second helpings.

Make good food choices

Don't grocery shop while hungry! Otherwise there is a risk you'll come home with fast food instead of a meal that takes time to cook.

Gradually replace high-calorie foods with fruit and vegetables. Switch to food with a low glycaemic index. This will make you feel full for longer and make you less hungry for the next meal, so you'll happily eat a small portion next time.

Drink water instead of beer and carbonated drinks.

Think twice before having a pastry

It can be eye-opening to see how much you need to exercise – walk briskly/jog – to burn off a particular type of food or drink. Note, however, that the figures in table 12 are approximate as they depend on how much you weigh and how you define a 'slice' of cake, for example.

Type of food or drink	Distance
• 1 cup of coffee, no sugar	0 km
• 150 ml low-alcohol beer	0.8 km
• 1 small cake	1.0 km
• 150 ml strong beer	1.4 km
• 150 ml wine	1.5 km
• 10 crisps	2 km
• 15 salted peanuts	2 km
• 10 French fries	4 km
• 1 Danish pastry	6 km
• 1 burger	8 km
• 1 tartlet	8 km
• 1 slice of cake	8 km
• 1 pizza	10 km

Table 12. How far you need to walk briskly/ jog to burn off types of food or drink

The figures above may be something to think about before you have a slice of cake or a pastry with your coffee!

MONITOR YOUR WEIGHT

When transforming your lifestyle and beginning to
think about a healthier weight, it is good to have a base
value to start with – what do the scales say? The scales
give immediate feedback about your current status
and whether you need to make any corrections in one
direction or the other. When you begin to change your
food choices and want to check your progress after
a few days, simply weigh yourself and you'll have an
answer on the spot – maybe a drop of 100 grams or
more. Encouraged by this, you can make further lifestyle
changes – and then check again. This way, you'll quickly
learn what you can eat and how you can live to keep
yourself at the weight you want.

If, at the same time, you start taking exercise, you'll gain
more muscle, which will actually increase your weight. In
this case your stomach measurement will provide a good
indication of how your abdominal fat is reducing and being
replaced by muscle instead. And all this will give you a
major boost towards better health!

If you don't monitor your progress, you might find yourself
eating and living in a way that allows your weight to
increase by a few hundred grams a week. If this continues
week after week, and happens so gradually that you don't

really notice it, suddenly you'll discover that you've gained 10 kg.

In keeping your weight in check, you can eat intelligently and well all your life, and fewer kilos may well translate into more years of life.

TOP TIPS

- Buy a good set of scales

- Weigh yourself as a matter of routine

- Quickly break any upward trend

- Keep a note of your weight – set a target

INTERMITTENT FASTING

A popular type of intermittent fasting is the 5:2 diet, which involves keeping your calorie intake very low for two days a week and eating normally on the other five days.

Another type of intermittent fast is the overnight fast, which means not eating between 6 pm one day and 12 noon the next.

Fasting has a positive effect on weight and diabetes, as well as lowering blood pressure, blood sugar and blood lipids (fats). During fasting, the body uses existing fat as a fuel source instead of sugar. This reduces the risk of both diabetes and cardiovascular disease.

TIP 8

• •

Oral health
gives general health

INFLAMMATION IN THE GUMS AFFECTS VASCULAR HEALTH

It has long been known that there is a strong link between cardiovascular disease and high blood pressure, smoking, stress, diabetes and obesity. There is also a correlation between poor oral health, smoking and poor food habits. But many people were surprised when a link began to emerge between gum inflammation around the teeth and diseases of the body's vascular system. How could oral health affect the health of our arteries?

Bleeding gums – a warning sign

It is known that gingivitis with bleeding gums often leads to deep periodontal pockets and, in the long run, tooth loss. Serious tooth decay can also cause inflammation in and around the teeth. If these dental diseases are left unchecked, ongoing inflammation of the gums can occur and this can cause bacteria to constantly spread through the blood vessels. This inflammation then affects not only the mouth but the whole body. The inflammation – which can last for weeks, months and years – damages the blood vessels, which can cause an increased risk of heart attack and stroke.

Research shows

A study revealed that people with gum disease and tooth decay had a mortality rate that was between just over 20 and almost 50 per cent higher than people without these diseases. This was accounted for by a higher incidence of cardiovascular disease and stroke.

Being free from gum disease is estimated to add more than six years to your life.

HOW CAN YOU PREVENT GUM DISEASE AND TOOTH DECAY?

Go to the dentist for regular check-ups. You can then usually halt dental diseases at an early stage with fewer or more minor treatments. The dentist will often also give individual advice on oral hygiene and diet.

Remember the 'two rule': brush your teeth with 2 cm of fluoride toothpaste for two minutes at least twice a day.

Cleaning between the teeth is as important as brushing and should also be done on a daily basis. Flossing may be more difficult for some than others, depending on how close together your teeth are. However, there are now all sorts of different toothpicks, dental flosses and interdental brushes that you can use. This is perhaps the most important thing you can do to prevent both gum disease and tooth decay, but it is also the easiest to forget. An advert encouraging the use of dental floss carried the following smart question and answer:

> **Question:** Which teeth should you floss between?
> **Answer:** Between the teeth you want to keep!

If you bear that in mind when you're standing in front of the bathroom mirror at night, you might feel more motivated not to skip flossing between any of your teeth! Instead, you can feel good about the fact that, by keeping your gums healthy, you are protecting yourself against inflammation in your entire body.

Avoid snacking between meals, eating sweets and similar treats since every time you eat, bacteria in the mouth breaks down sugar into acid that can burn holes in the tooth enamel. After every consumption of sugar – large or small – the acid state will last for thirty minutes. If your sugar intake amounts to just one sweet six times a day, your teeth could be exposed to acid for three hours in total! This can cause tooth decay and, over time, inflamed gums.

Many medicines cause a dry mouth as a side effect and this can reduce resistance to dental diseases. Rinsing your mouth with water is an easy and effective way to relieve symptoms. You can also buy lozenges or mouth spray at the pharmacy.

TIP 9

• • • • • • • • • • • • • • • • • • • •

Be an optimist

The question of whether you see the glass as half full or half empty is a simple indication of how you look at life – optimistically or pessimistically. The optimist has the positive thought 'how great that there is still half left' while the pessimist focuses on the negative: 'it'll soon be all gone'. This attitude to life is highly significant when it comes to impacts on health. Not only does the optimist live longer, he/she also has better attention levels, a better memory, more curiosity, makes friends more easily, has more success at work and a more enjoyable life. Feeling hope and optimism is an important factor in feeling well. We are born with a drive not just to survive, but to live.

WHY DO OPTIMISTS LIVE LONGER?

The optimist is solution-driven, while the pessimist is problem-oriented. When problems or setbacks occur, optimists put their energy into 'how can I resolve this' and visualise success. This sidesteps feelings of stress, frustration and powerlessness, and thus avoids higher blood sugar levels, increased inflammation and damage to the immune system. This in turn stems the development of cancer and cardiovascular disease. Pessimists, on the other hand, channel their energy into worrying and getting stressed, which causes increased inflammation and premature death.

● ●

Research shows

A study of 5,000 adults examined the participants' cardiovascular status and their level of optimism. The results showed that those with a positive view of life were twice as likely to have good heart health, compared with those who had a negative view of life. The optimists had better blood sugar and blood lipid (fat) levels.

One study followed over 120 men who had recently suffered their first heart attack. Eight years later, twenty-one of the twenty-five most pessimistic men had died, while only six of the twenty-five most optimistic men had died.

Of those who die prematurely, seven out of ten are pessimists.

● ●

Optimists live longer than pessimists, with studies showing a difference of up to seven years.

WHAT CHARACTERISES THE OPTIMIST AND THE PESSIMIST?

An *optimist* always sees a solution to every problem.
A *pessimist* finds a problem in every solution.

An *optimist* says – I can if I want.
A *pessimist* says – I can't do it, I might as well give up.

An *optimist* says – it's difficult, yes, but possible.
A *pessimist* says – this might be possible but it's far too difficult.

An *optimist* says – what lovely weather, the sun is shining.
A *pessimist* says – today it is, but . . .

The *optimist* creates better times.
The *pessimist* waits for better times.

CAN YOU BECOME AN OPTIMIST AND IF SO HOW?

Create motivation

If you lean towards pessimism, it can be a good health strategy to try and change your attitude to life. Nobody is born a pessimist, you become one. We can learn to be unhappy and some people practise it every day!

But we can also learn optimism and hope. However, it is not easy once you have settled into certain patterns of thought and behaviour. To break this pattern, you have to be motivated to change. Thinking about the benefits – getting to live perhaps seven years longer and healthier, having more friends and having more fun than before – could be a good driver of change.

Start with self-awareness

Take a step back. Study yourself and your reactions, be self-critical, feel when the pessimism begins to flow. Listen to yourself when you talk about the misery in your life and the wider world, about everything that makes you angry, sad and disappointed. Gain an awareness of how much energy you put into things that are negative or are not going to go well.

Create positive images

Try instead to see everything from a different angle and try to think and act in a new way. Use your energy to create positive pictures of what you have to be thankful for, what makes you happy and what you enjoy. This is where the optimism journey begins.

Think positively – in the right way

There is a wealth of power in being able to think positively. Say positive things and feed the brain with positive messages. But this doesn't mean you should become a dreamer with masses of unrealistic goals. An optimistic, realistic person who uses the power of thought correctly is rooted in reality and sees difficulties and problems, but they rarely let them get them down. The optimist doesn't try to ignore the negative but is not confined by it and always works to change and convert the negative into something positive. The optimist hopes for the best, but is prepared for the worst.

Express gratitude and joy

Acknowledge what is meaningful in your life and embrace everything around you that is good. Express gratitude and joy for the big things and the small. What this generates is a general level of 'everyday happiness'. The optimist sees this and it fills them with positive emotions.

Surround yourself with positive people

You are who you spend time with. Avoid pessimists who drain your energy. Instead, socialise in circles where the optimists can be found. They radiate energy – it's infectious. Then share your positive energy with your nearest and dearest. This will create *joie de vivre* and health for both you and those around you.

Laugh and smile

Humour and laughter reduce stress hormones, lower blood pressure and improve your mood. Laughing increases the level of endorphins, which gives a feeling of pleasure and reward. Feelings of stress disappear, inflammation in the body reduces and the immune system becomes stronger and more effective. There really is something in the old saying that 'laughter is the best medicine'. Act like a happy person, walk around with a spring in your step and a smile on your lips and this will cheer you up.

Be physically active

Physical activity of various kinds burns up stress hormones and releases the feel-good hormone dopamine. This creates a sense of well-being that makes it easier to think positive thoughts.

Be generous towards others

At heart, people are givers and we get more pleasure from giving than from receiving. So give your energy and time freely. If you are in the habit of giving a helping hand to someone who needs it, of being there for a friend, that is an important source of positive feelings. Be just as enthusiastic about other people's successes as you are about your own.

TIP 10

· · · · · · · · · · · · · · · · · · · ·

We need each other

• • • • • • • • • • • • • • • • • • • •

People are pack animals, we need each other. There is
a deep-seated need for social relationships and human
support in order to survive and stay healthy. Social
intercourse may well have been one of the key strategies for
the survival of the human race.

At the heart of a harmonious existence lie good family
relationships, work colleagues and a stable circle of friends.
But it is not the number of friends and social encounters
that is important, it is their quality. Good relationships
with a few are better than many relationships of poor
quality.

You can feel alone even when you are surrounded by
people, either in a couple or a group. Everyone is alone
sometimes and it is normal to feel lonely. Self-imposed
solitude is not associated with any health risk. The problem
is with involuntary loneliness.

THE DANGERS OF LONELINESS

If social relationships are insufficient over a prolonged period, the vulnerability of the individual increases. The dangers of loneliness arise from not having anyone to share your feelings with or to have close contact with. Loneliness can cause more suffering than physical pain.

Sometimes those around you help to make the loneliness feel even worse. One example is the elated grandmother who talks and talks about her fantastic children, not to mention her even more incredible grandchildren. She doesn't think for a second that there may be someone listening in the group who doesn't have any family or whose childlessness was not a choice. It is therefore important to be aware of the situation you are in and to think about what you say, so as not to hurt anyone. It is also important to be on the lookout for anyone, for example at work, who feels excluded from the social group. In such a case it is good to be generous, to show engagement with and interest in the person in question, invite them for a chat – and see a friendship develop.

Our social environment has crucial consequences for our health. If you feel lonely, excluded and without support, your resistance to stress and disease is reduced. Psychological stress creates inflammation and has a direct harmful effect on the immune system, the cardiovascular system and the body's other organs. This raises the risk of illness and a shorter life.

Many people are well aware that stress, obesity and sitting still are harmful to health, but it is much less well known that involuntary loneliness can be a major factor in ill health. The advice in this chapter therefore delves more deeply into ways of shaking off loneliness, something that is largely an internal process.

The dangers of loneliness double the risk of falling ill and dying. Feeling excluded affects mortality just as much as – or more than – smoking, stress, obesity or high blood pressure.

WHAT DO YOU GAIN FROM TIME WITH FRIENDS?

Everything that promotes feelings of inclusion and social belonging and that makes you feel respected and liked for who you are – and being able to give the same back – is good for you. The more we share with each other, the healthier and stronger we and our relationships are.

A good social life has a positive effect in that it boosts the feel-good hormone, reduces the stress hormones and thereby also decreases inflammation. Our immune system is strengthened and this leads to a longer life, with more fun in it.

You may be strong on your own, but being part of a positive social circle makes you even stronger.

Those who live in positive relationships – with good, close relatives, friends or a beloved pet – recover faster from illness and live longer.

● ●

Research shows

Several studies have shown higher mortality among individuals who are lonely. For example, a person living alone has a higher risk of dying from a stroke than people living together.

In a large study of 180,000 people, the risk of a heart attack rose by almost 30 per cent in those who felt lonely or had few social contacts. The corresponding figure for stroke was an increased risk of just over 30 per cent.

A US study showed that the risk of developing Alzheimer's was more than twice as great for those who felt lonely, compared with those who didn't.

● ●

THE KEY TO CHANGE

Step one: understanding

The first step is to understand your situation, be honest with yourself, clearly see the problem and understand its consequences.

'I'm lonely, I don't have any really good friends or a life partner, I sit here all alone on a Friday night, while others have cosy evenings together. The big holidays are the saddest days of the year, when the loneliness is particularly painful. I'm often sad and it feels like life is just passing me by.'

It can be tough to put together this picture of yourself and really understand your situation. But this is how you enable change, as in this moment of clarity you may realise that something has to be done.

Step two: create motivation

And so the ideas come quickly about maybe trying something new. This creates motivation and that is the wave of energy that will lead you to take action to break the cycle of loneliness.

Each individual will usually have their own solution to the problem – something that suits their particular situation. The best solution is there – inside yourself.

In this phase, you have to overcome your fears: 'What if I embarrass myself? What if something happens to me as I walk home in the dark? What if I get tricked by someone on social media?' Fear is a defence mechanism that can make life very limited. But now you have to let go, dare to move on. You should still be critically assessing the various alternatives, but don't exaggerate the dangers. Instead, paint a positive picture of what you want to achieve.

Step three: set a goal

You now have the motivation and drive to change your situation and so you need to immediately set your goal: 'What do I want my life to look like and how can I achieve that? What do I need to do first? What should I try?' Now you're on the right track – a goal has been set and a decision made.

Step four: take the initiative

And now for action – finally there is a chance of something happening. Naturally, there are friends or a good partner out there for you, you just need the energy and the focus to find the 'treasure' – because having friends and leading a longer, healthier and more fun life truly is a treasure.

DEVELOP FRIENDSHIPS

Developing friendship takes time and good friendship has to be nurtured and maintained. You have to care, make contact and listen. The friendship will then deepen over time and become a source of joy and trust. To establish a good relationship with other people, it is important to:

- Speak from the heart, be able to talk about topics large and small, be a good listener.

- Be positive, show appreciation, give feedback, have fun together.

- Respect each other's differences, be able to compromise and be flexible.

When it comes to that wonderful, genuine meeting between people, it is important to feel and show empathy – to always try to put yourself in the other person's shoes. If you don't know where he/she is coming from, you can't properly be a good friend and show mutual respect. Nor can you give support or advice if the need arises. Keeping this in mind as you develop your network of close friends will make those friendships deep, lasting and enriching.

HOW DO YOU FIND NEW FRIENDS?

Friendships can be created in many different ways and they don't have to be age-dependent. Friends of different ages make life richer. Everyone has opportunities to find new friends, whatever their situation.

Contacts can be made by:

- Attending a course or joining a club that interests you, for example a cookery course, photography course, birdwatching, a gardening club, sports club – where you'll meet like-minded people.

- Having the courage to travel alone and talk to people you don't know.

- Going out dancing.

- Using social media such as Facebook, chat rooms, online dating sites.

- Taking up walking, exercise or going to the gym with someone.

- Inviting a neighbour round for tea or coffee, or going to the cinema with someone.

- Getting involved in community organisations.

- Singing in a choir.

- Having a beloved pet as a friend.

MAKING FRIENDS ISN'T EASY

There are all sorts of obstacles that can stop making contact with others from happening. The most common of these are:

- Fear: the prospect of meeting new people can be both exciting and terrifying. Fear often wins out over curiosity.

- Low self-esteem: 'Why would anyone want to spend time with me? I have nothing to offer and everyone is bound to find me boring.'

- An unsafe neighbourhood and fear of going out alone at night. This can stop you going out and meeting people.

Fear and low self-esteem lead people to make poor decisions. Despite being unhappy about the loneliness, they can't pluck up the courage to do anything about it.

AVOID ENERGY THIEVES

Good relationships create positive energy that promotes health and well-being. However, the opposite is also true, with some people around you stealing your energy. After such an encounter, you can feel tired, drained and a bit of a failure. Choose the right friends and foster a healthy social life.

DON'T GIVE UP

If anxiety and insecurity arise, take stock of your current situation. 'This is what my life is like today – do I want to keep living this way?' The answer is no – so embrace your vision again and overcome the fear – it's time for things to start happening. Don't think 'How is it going to go?' but 'What must I do to make it go well?'

There are plenty of lovely little cards available with sayings and messages about daring to take the first step, believing in yourself, you can do it, you are worth it and so on.

These affirmations can be placed on the bathroom mirror or the fridge, for example, as a reminder of this new self-image and that you are going to succeed.

Once you've taken a first step, you've set things in motion and then it's easy to think, 'Now I'm going to take the next step.' It becomes a positive spiral, after that most difficult first step.

Of course there will be days when you start to doubt yourself and feel tired and vulnerable. Maybe that day you won't take a step forward, but it is important to keep your goal in mind and get started again as soon as possible. Don't give up at the first hurdle, instead maybe try being even more flexible about the way you achieve your goal. If your first attempt doesn't go well, think of a new, possibly better, solution.

If a setback can be seen as a valuable and important experience, this increases the chance of things going better next time. Setbacks are good as they offer an opportunity to grow and develop. An unwillingness to fail comes down to fear. But let your curiosity prevail instead. Uncertainty is part of life, the part that makes it exciting. Spread your wings, dare to succeed!

Conclusion

• • • • • • • • • • • • • • • • • • • •

This book may have come to an end, but the rest of your life has just begun! How are you going to live it? Now you know what makes you stronger and what slows the ageing process.

You have the chance to change your lifestyle, so my final tip is: start today – or tomorrow!

Good luck!

Facts and references

● ● ● ● ● ● ● ● ● ● ● ● ● ● ● ● ● ● ●

The book's facts are all based on the knowledge and experience that I have gained from my twenty years as a doctor in primary care and then twenty years as a researcher into general medicine and public health at the University of Gothenburg.

The book's facts are also based on a large number of scientific articles, systematic summaries of research results, reference books, national guidelines and statements by established and respected researchers and authors.

Bibliography

General references with links to multiple chapters in the book:

Antonovsky A., *Hälsans Mysterium*, 2nd edition,
    Stockholm: Natur och Kultur; 2005 (*Unravelling the
    mystery of health*, Jossey-Bass Inc, Publishers 1987).
Carper J., *Mirakelhjärnan* (*The Miracle Brain*), 2nd
    edition, Stockholm: Forum; 2001.
Csíkszentmihályi M. *Finna Flow, den vardagliga
    entusiasmens psykologi* (*Find flow, the psychology of
    everyday enthusiasm*), Stockholm: Natur och Kultur;
    1999.
Ehdin Anandala S., *Nya självläkande människan* (*The new
    self-healing human*), 2nd edition, Bladh by Bladh;
    2014.
Ennart H., *Åldrandets gåta, metoderna som förlänger ditt
    liv* (*The riddle of ageing, methods that extend your
    life*), Stockholm: Ordfront; 2013.
Marklund B., *Symtom, Råd, Åtgärd* (*Symptoms, Advice,
    Action*), 9th edition, Studentlitteratur; 2008.
Roizen M., *Real Age. Are you as young as you can be?*,
    Harper Collins e-books; 2010.
Servan-Schreiber D., *Anticancer, ett nytt sätt att leva*
    (*Anticancer: a new way of living*), Stockholm: Natur
    och Kultur; 2011.
World Health Organisation, 'The Ottawa Charter for
    Health Promotion', WHO Regional Office for Europe:
    Copenhagen; 1986.

Specific references with links to particular chapters in the
book:

What determines the length of your life?

Khaw, K., et al., 'Combined impact of health behaviours and mortality in men and women', the EPIC-Norfolk prospective population study, *PlosMedicine*; 5, 39–47; e12, 2008.

Knoops, K.T.B., et al., 'Mediterranean diet, lifestyle factors and 10-year mortality in elderly European men and women: the HALE Project', *JAMA*; 292:1433–1439; 2004.

Lichtenstein, P., Holm N.V., Verkasalo P.K., et al., 'Environmental and heritable factors in the causation of cancer – Analyses of cohorts of twins from Sweden, Denmark, and Finland', *New England Journal of Medicine*; 343:78–85; 2000.

Wilhelmsen L., Svärdsudd K., Eriksson H., et al., 'Factors associated with reaching 90 years of age; a study of men born in 1913 in Gothenburg, Sweden', *Journal of Internal Medicine*; 269:441–451; 2011.

Movement rejuvenates the body

Biswas A., Paul I., Faulkner G., et al., 'Sedentary time and its association with risk for disease incidence, mortality, and hospitalization in adults: A systematic review and meta-analysis', *Annals of Internal Medicine*; 162:123–132; 2015.

Dunstan D.W., Barr E.L., Healy G.N., et al., 'Television viewing time and mortality: the Australian Diabetes, Obesity and Lifestyle Study', *Circulation*; 121:384–391; 2010.

Fröberg A., Raustorp A., 'Samband mellan stillasittande och ohälsa varierar med mätmetod' ('Correlation between sitting still and ill-health varies with measurement method'), *Läkartidningen*; 113:DU33; 2016.

Henriksson J., Ekbom M., Tranquist J., 'FYSS: Fysisk aktivitet i sjukdomsprevention och sjukdomsbehandling' ('Physical activity in disease prevention and disease treatment'), Swedish National Institute of Public Health; 2003.

Jansson E., Hagströmer M., Anderssen S., 'Fysisk aktivitet – nya vägar och val i rekommendationerna för vuxna' ('Physical activity – new paths and options in recommendations for adults'), *Läkartidningen*; 112:DP7W; 2015.

Johansson S., Qvist J., 'Motion förlänger livet' ('Exercise extends life'), *Välfärdsbulletinen*; 2:12; 1997.

Norling I., Sullivan M., Marklund B., 'Fritid och hälsa' ('Recreation and health'), Report 11, Gothenburg; 1995.

Senchina D.S., 'Effects of regular exercise on the aging immune system: a review', *Clinical Journal of Sport Medicine*; 19:439–440; 2009.

Smith T.C., 'Walking decreased risk of cardiovascular disease mortality in older adults with diabetes', *Journal of Clinical Epidemiology*; 60:309–317; 2007.

Sundberg C. J., Jansson E., 'Fysisk aktivitet en viktig medicin' ('Physical activity an important medicine'), *Läkartidningen*; 112:DRT4; 2015.

Time for recovery

Arnetz B, Ekman R. (ed), *Stress. Gen Individ Samhälle* (*Stress. Gene Individual Society*), 3rd edition: Liber AB; 2013.

Kivipelto M., et al., 'A 2-year multidomain intervention of diet, exercise, cognitive training, and vascular risk monitoring versus control to prevent cognitive decline in at-risk elderly people (FINGER): a randomised controlled trial', *Lancet*; 385:2255–2263; 2015.

Melander O., Melander M.O., Manjer J., et al., 'Stable peptide of the endogenous opioid enkephalin precursor and breast cancer risk', *Journal of Clinical Oncology*; 33:2632–38; 2015.

Sleep fortifies

Bellavia A., Åkerstedt T., Bottai M., et al., 'Sleep duration and survival percentiles across categories of physical activity', *American Journal of Epidemiology*; 179:484–491; 2014.

Kripke D., Garfinkel L., Deborah L., et al., 'Mortality associated with sleep duration and insomnia FREE', *Archives of General Psychiatry*; 59:131–136; 2002.

Naska A., Oikonomous E., Trichopoulou A. et al., 'Siesta in healthy adults and coronary mortality in the general population', *Archives of Internal Medicine*; 167:296–301; 2007.

Åkerstedt T., 'Livsstilen påverkar sömnen – på gott och ont' ('Lifestyle affects sleep – for good and bad'), *Läkartidningen*; 107:2072–2076; 2010.

Sun – but not too much

Giovannucci E., Speech at the American Association for Cancer Research conference in Arnaheim, California; 2005.

Giovannucci E., 'Vitamin D status and cancer incidence and mortality', *Advances in Experimental Medicine and Biology*; 624:31–42; 2008.

Lindqvist P.G., Epstein E., Nielsen K., et al., 'Avoidance of sun exposure as a risk factor for major causes of death: a competing risk analysis of the melanoma in southern Sweden cohort', *Journal of Internal Medicine*; 280:375–387; 2016.

National Health Service UK, Vitamins and Minerals – Vitamin D. http://www.nhs.uk/Conditions/vitamins-minerals/Pages/Vitamin-D.aspx.

Tuohimaa P., Pukkala E., Scélo G., et al., 'Does solar exposure, as indicated by the non-melanoma skin cancers, protect from solid cancers: Vitamin D as a possible explanation', *European Journal of Cancer*; 43:1701–1712; 2007.

Eat yourself healthy

BBC Good Food Nation, 2015. Immediate Media Co. press release. http://www.immediate.co.uk/news/brand/nearly-two-thirds-of-population-do-not-eat-5-a-day-indicates-bbc-good-food-study/

Bengmark S., 'Vår tids kost bakom inflammation och sjukdomsutveckling' ('Modern diet behind inflammation and disease development'), *Läkartidningen*; 104:3873–3877; 2007.

Bengmark S., 'Den bioekologiska medicinen har kommit för att stanna. Om flora, synbiotika, immunitet och resistens mot sjukdom' ('Bioecological medicine is here to stay. On flora, synbiotics, immunity and resistance to disease'), *Läkartidningen*; 102:2–6; 2005.

Cederholm T., Hellénius M.-L., 'Matens betydelse för åldrande och livslängd', ('The importance of nutrition in healthy ageing and longevity'), *Läkartidningen*; 113:DYMA; 2016.

Cederholm T., Rothenberg E., 'Krypskytte mot vetenskapen äventyrar folkhälsoarbetet' ('Sniping against science jeopardises public health work'), *Läkartidningen*; 113:784–785; 2016.

Knoops K.T., de Groot L.C., Kromhout D., et al., 'Mediterranean diet, lifestyle factors, and 10-year mortality in elderly European men and women: the HALE project', *JAMA*; 292:1433–1439; 2004.

Kwok C.S., Boekholdt M., Lentjes M., et al., 'Habitual chocolate consumption and risk of cardiovascular disease among healthy men and women', *Heart*, epub 15 June 2015. doi:10.1136/heartjnl-2014-307050.

Lindstedt I., Nilsson P., 'Flavanoler, kakao och choklad påverkar hjärt- kärlsystemet' ('Flavanols, cocoa and chocolate affect the cardiovascular system'), *Läkartidningen*; 108:324–325; 2011.

Liu S. et al., 'Whole-grain consumption and risk of coronary heart disease: results from the Nurses' Health Study', *American Journal of Clinical Nutrition*; 70:412–419; 1999.

National Health Service, Fish and shellfish. http://www.nhs.uk/Livewell/Goodfood/Pages/fish-shellfish.aspx.

National Health Service, Red meat and the risk of bowel cancer. http://www.nhs.uk/Livewell/Goodfood/Pages/red-meat.aspx.

Nilsson P.M., 'Medelhavskosten skyddar hjärtat' ('Mediterranean diet protects the heart'),

Läkartidningen; 106:1959; 2009.

'Nordic Nutrition Recommendations 2012. Integrating nutrition and physical activity', 5th edition: Copenhagen: Nordic Council of Ministers; Nord 2014:002; 2014.

Paulun F., 'Blodsockerblues – en bok om glykemiskt index' ('Blood sugar blues – a book about the glycaemic index'), *Fitnessförlaget*, 2003.

Rydén L., Andersen K., Gyberg V., et al., 'Betala för sjukdom eller investera i hälsa?' ('Pay for disease or invest in health?'), *Läkartidningen*; 109:1535–1539; 2012.

Simopoulos A., 'Importance of the omega-6/omega-3 balance in health and disease: Evolutionary aspects of diet', *World Review of Nutrition and Dietetics*: Basel, Karger; 102:10–21; 2011.

Stender S., Astrup A., Dyerberg J., 'Ruminant and industrially produced trans fatty acids: health aspects', *Food and Nutrition Research*; 2008. DOI: 10.3402/fnr.v52i0.1651.

Stender S., Astrup A., Dyerberg J., 'Tracing artificial trans fat in popular foods in Europe: a market basket investigation', *BMJ Open*; 4; 2014. e.005218.

Swedish National Food Agency, Dietary advice and food habits, 2015.

Wolk A., Bergström R., Hunder H., et al., 'A prospective study of association of monosaturated fat and other types of fat with risk of breast cancer FREE', *Archives of Internal Medicine*; 158:41–45; 1998.

World Cancer Research Fund International, Continuous Update Project; September 2015.

Choose the right drink

Bhupathiraju S.N., Manson J.E., Willett W.C., et al., 'Changes in coffee intake and subsequent risk of type 2 diabetes: three large cohorts of US men and women', *Diabetologia*; 57:1346–1354; 2014.

Department of Health, UK Chief Medical Officers' Alcohol Guidelines Review, https://www.gov.uk/government/uploads/system/uploads/attachment_data/file/489795/summary.pdf.

Eskelinen H.H., Ngandu T., Tuomilehto J., et al., 'Midlife coffee and tea drinking and the risk of late-life dementia: a population-based CAIDE study', *Journal of Alzheimer's Disease*; 16:85–91; 2009.

Fagrell B., Hultcrantz R., 'Alkohol inte enbart av ondo – måttligt intag minskar risk för folksjukdomar' ('Alcohol not just bad – moderate consumption reduces the risk of common diseases'), *Läkartidningen*; 109:1884–1888; 2012.

Fredholm B., 'Kaffe minskar risk för Parkinsons sjukdom' ('Coffee reduces the risk of Parkinson's disease'), *Läkartidningen*; 101:2552–2556; 2004.

Guercio B.J., Sato K., Niedzwiecki D., et al., 'Coffee intake, recurrence, and mortality in stage III colon cancer', *Journal of Clinical Oncology*, 31: 3598–3607; 2015.

Hansen A., 'Kaffe minskar risken för stroke' ('Coffee reduces the risk of stroke'), *Läkartidningen*; 106: 919; 2009.

Rosendahl A., Perks C., Zeng L., et al., 'Caffeine and caffeic acid inhibit growth and modify estrogen receptor and insulin-like growth factor I receptor levels in human breast cancer', *Clinical Cancer Research*; 21:1877-87; 2015.

Keep your weight in check

Bengmark B., 'Obesity, the deadly quartet and the contribution of the neglected daily organ rest – a new dimension on un-health and its prevention', *HepatoBiliary Surgery and Nutrition*; 4:278–288; 2015.

Läkemedelsboken, Swedish Medical Products Agency, *Overweight and Obesity*, 201–208; 2014.

Oral health gives general health

Hugosson A., et al., 'Oral health of individuals aged 3–80 years in Jönköping, Sweden during 30 years (1973–2003) II'. Review of clinical and radiographic findings. *Swedish Dental Journals*; 29:139–155; 2005.

Hugosson A., Norderyd O., Slotte C., et al., 'Distribution of periodontology disease in a Swedish adult population 1973, 1983 and 1993', *Journal of Clinical Peridontology*; 25:542–548; 1998.

Vedin O., 'Prevalence and prognostic impact of peridontal disease and conventional risk factors in patients with stable coronary heart disease', thesis, Uppsala University; 2015.

Be an optimist

Chida Y. Steptoe A., 'Positive psychological well-being and mortality: A quantitative review of prospective observational studies', *Psychosomatic Medicine*; 70:741–756; 2008.

Fexeus H., 'Konsten att få superkrafter' ('The art of gaining superpowers'), Stockholm: Forum; pp 396–398; 2012.

Hernandez R., Kershaw K., Siddique J., et al., 'Optimism and cardiovascular health: Multi-ethnic study of atherosclerosis (MESA)', *Health Behaviour & Policy Review*; 2:62–73; 2015.

Sebö, S., 'Bruksanvisning för ett bättre Liv' ('Instructions for a better life'), edition 2.2: Uppsala; Konsultförlaget; 2000.

We need each other

Cole S., Capitanio J., Chun K., et al., 'Myeloid differential architecture of leukocyte transcriptome dynamics in perceived social isolation'. Proceedings of the National Academy of Science of the United States of America. 112:15142–47; 2015.

Lindmark A., Glader E.L., Asplund K., et al., 'Socioeconomic disparities in stroke case fatality – observations from Riks-Stroke, the Swedish stroke register', *International Journal of Stroke*; 9:429–436; 2014.

Valtora N.K., et al., 'Loneliness and social isolation as risk factors for coronary heart disease and stroke: systemic review and meta-analysis of longitudinal observational studies', *Heart*: epub 19 March 2016.

Wilson R.S., et al., 'Loneliness and risk of Alzheimer disease', *Archives of General Psychiatry*; 64:234–240; 2007.

Thanks

• • • • • • • • • • • • • • • • • • •

I have received invaluable feedback on this book from:

Johan Appel, Tina Arvidsdotter, Harald Arvidsson, Jenny
Bernson, Maria Fredriksson, Sven Kylén, Eva Larsson,
Johan Malmquist, Åsa Marklund, Håkan Patrikson and
family members Karin, Martin and Ola Marklund.

I would also like to thank my daughter Karin Marklund
and journalist Nina Olsson for their superb proofreading
of the whole text. Thanks also go to my sister, Britt-Inger
Henrikson PhD, for her professional review of the scientific
rigour in the book.

Last but not least, I would like to thank Jillian Young at
Piatkus and Christine Edhäll at Ahlander Agency for an
excellent collaboration and for their fantastic work on this
book.

Bertil Marklund, Vänersborg

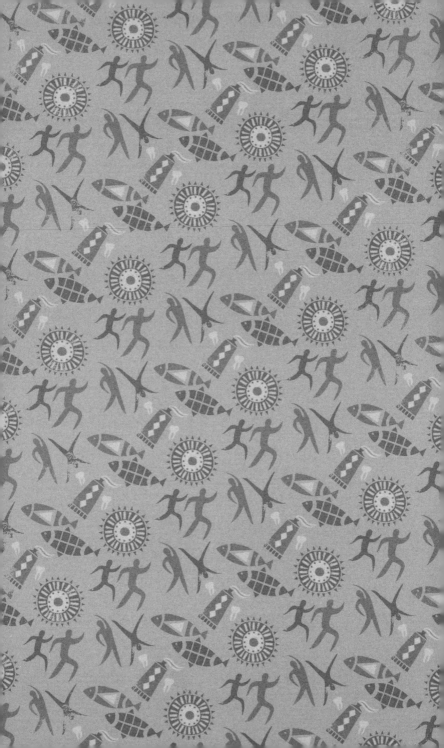